Pneumothorax

Edited by Khalid Amer

Published in London, United Kingdom

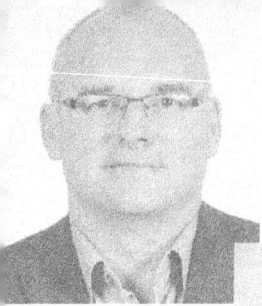
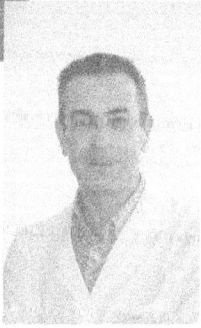
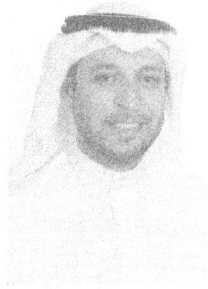
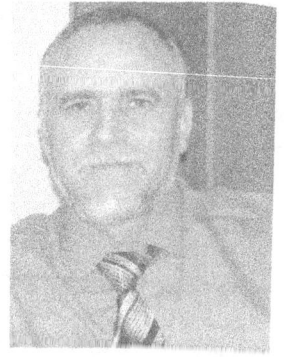
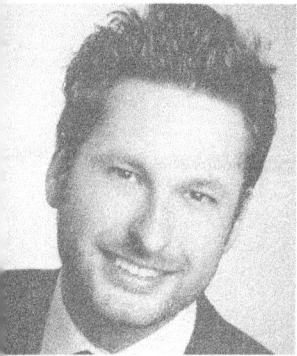
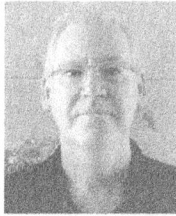
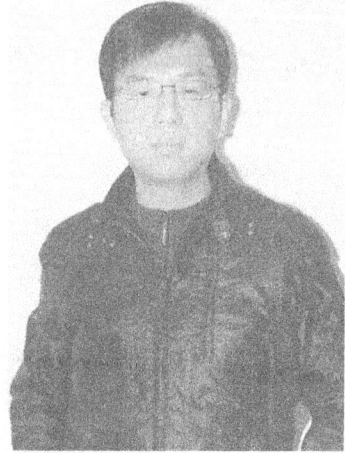

IntechOpen

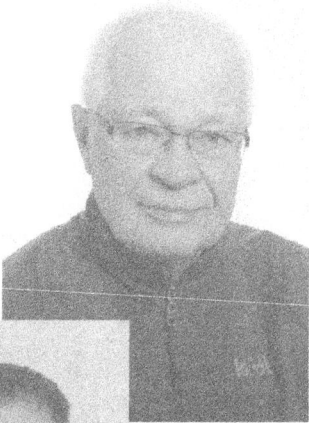
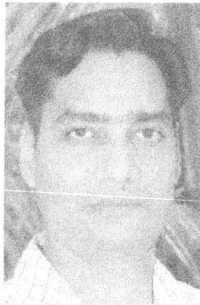
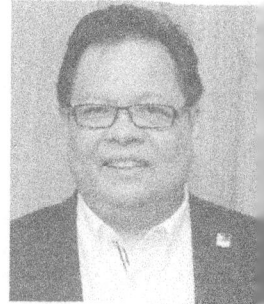
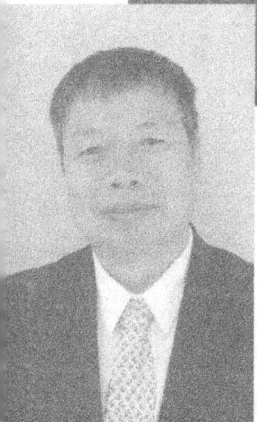
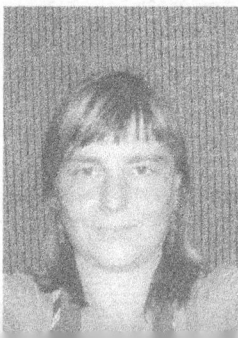
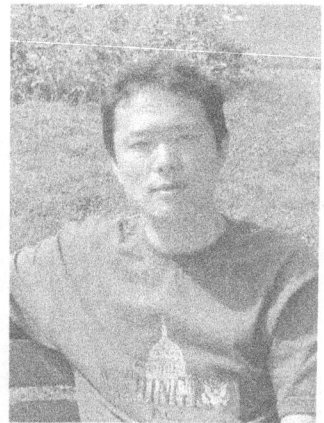

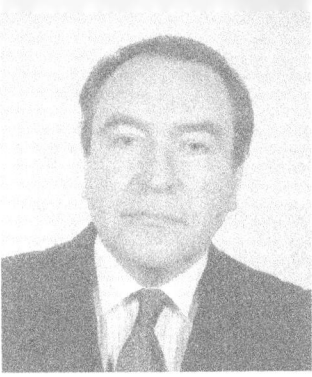

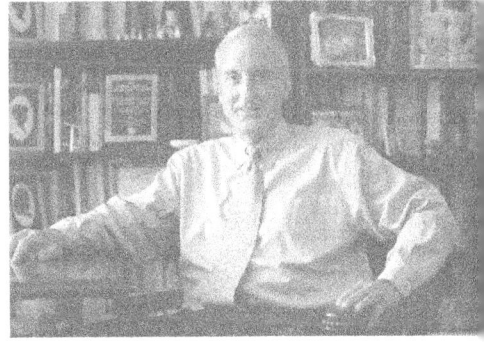

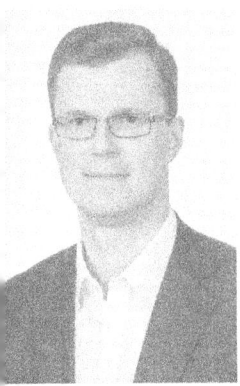

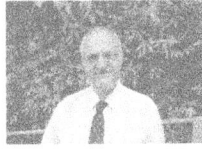

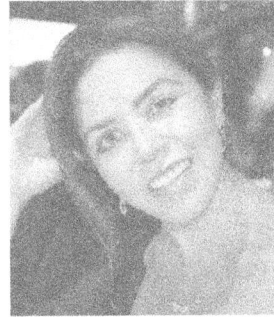

Supporting open minds since 2005

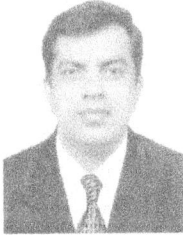

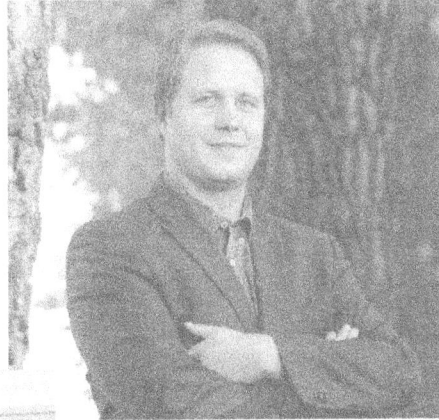

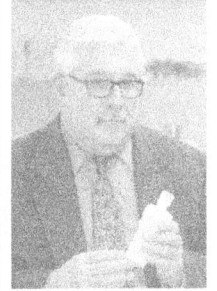

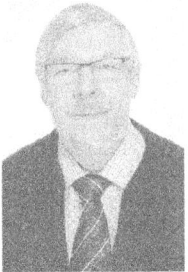

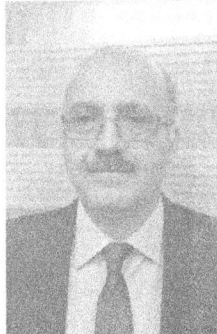

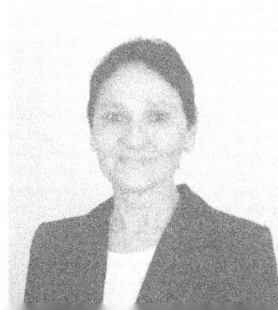

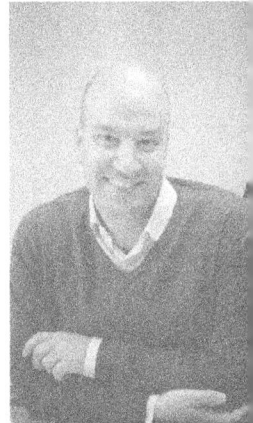

Pneumothorax
http://dx.doi.org/10.5772/intechopen.73885
Edited by Khalid Amer

Contributors
Fabian Giraldo, Ruby Romero, Melissa Mejia, Estefania Quijano, Wickii Vigneswaran, John Costello, Kostantinos Poulikidis, Lee Gerson, Sezai Celik, Ezel Erşen, Hany Hasan Elsayed, Khalid Amer

Notice
Statements and opinions expressed in the chapters are these of the individual contributors and not necessarily those of the editors or publisher. No responsibility is accepted for the accuracy of information contained in the published chapters. The publisher assumes no responsibility for any damage or injury to persons or property arising out of the use of any materials, instructions, methods or ideas contained in the book.

First published in London, United Kingdom, 2019 by IntechOpen
IntechOpen is the global imprint of INTECHOPEN LIMITED, registered in England and Wales, registration number: 11086078, 7th floor, 10 Lower Thames Street, London,
EC3R 6AF, United Kingdom
Printed in Croatia

British Library Cataloguing-in-Publication Data
A catalogue record for this book is available from the British Library

Additional hard and PDF copies can be obtained from orders@intechopen.com

Pneumothorax
Edited by Khalid Amer
p. cm.
Print ISBN 978-1-83968-065-6
Online ISBN 978-1-83968-066-3
eBook (PDF) ISBN 978-1-83968-067-0

We are IntechOpen,
the world's leading publisher of
Open Access books

Built by scientists, for scientists

4,500+

Open access books available

118,000+

International authors and editors

130M+

Downloads

Our authors are among the

151

Countries delivered to

Top 1%

most cited scientists

12.2%

Contributors from top 500 universities

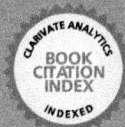

Interested in publishing with us?
Contact book.department@intechopen.com

Numbers displayed above are based on latest data collected.
For more information visit www.intechopen.com

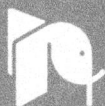

Meet the editor

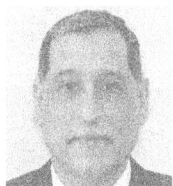

Dr. Amer was educated at Khartoum, Sudan, and studied medicine at the University of Khartoum. He obtained an MD degree in general surgery from the University of Khartoum before immigrating to the United Kingdom in 1992. He obtained the FRCS (en) in 1994 and started a training program in cardiothoracic surgery for six years at the University Hospital of Wales, Cardiff. He was certified in 2000 as a fellow of the four Royal Colleges in cardiothoracic surgery. He worked as a locum consultant cardiac surgeon for 3 years before his appointment as a pure thoracic surgeon in 2003 at Southampton General Hospital. Since then he has dedicated his career to video-assisted thoracic surgery. He was the founder of the VATS Programme at Southampton, and has since contributed to pushing the envelope of VATS to find new indications for the procedure. His seminal work is in VATS mediastinal nodal dissection and anatomy of the recurrent laryngeal nerves in the chest.

Contents

Preface

Having spent nearly 25 years in the specialty of Cardiothoracic Surgery in the UK, one would have thought that managing pneumothorax should come as a second nature. It doesn't. Humans collapse their lungs frequently, and the different ways we deal with this complication matches its frequency. There are bound to be differences in opinion, and the multicentre randomized controlled trials have not come up with a solid protocol to guide management. During my years of training as a cardiothoracic surgeon, I worked for several consultants, without any two of them agreeing on the management of this condition. Jean-Marc Gaspard Itard, a student of René Laennec's, first recognized the entity of the pneumothorax in 1803, but it was Laennec who described the full clinical picture of the condition in 1819 [1]. There was no general agreement on therapy when Ruckley and McCormac of the Royal Infirmary, Edinburgh described the management of pneumothorax in 1966 [2]. There is no agreement at our present time either. Robert Cerfolio summarized the conflict in few words; "although thoracic surgeons are the best trained physicians to manage chest tubes and pleural problems, they often do not speak the same language or recommend similar treatment algorithms even to each other" [3]. This sentiment inspired the collation of all information about "pneumothorax" under one roof. We aimed it at clinicians who encounter pneumothorax in their practice; pulmonologists, thoracic surgeons, pediatricians, obstetricians, and intensivists looking after sick ventilated patients in the Intensive Care Units amongst other clinicians. Based on published evidence, the book describes evidence and contemporary management of primary and secondary pneumothorax, when to adopt conservative management for first time primary pneumothorax and when to abandon it for surgical solutions. The evidence is discussed for and against key hole and open operations. Strategies for special circumstances are discussed, such as pneumothorax around menstrual cycles, during pregnancy, and before general anesthesia for other reasons, air travel, and scuba diving. A separate chapter highlights the current controversies about the different modalities of treatment. This is a book for every clinician struggling to find evidence on the best practice, and lost among the different contradicting rules and taboos of current practice. Further research remains the only way forward to narrow down our choices for what to do in the different scenarios of "pneumothorax".

Mr. Khalid M A Amer
FRCS (C Th) [Fellow of the Four Royal Colleges of Surgery Cardio Thoracic]
FRCS (en) [Fellow of the Royal College of Surgeons – England]
MD Clinical Surgery – University of Khartoum,
Sudan

Consultant Thoracic Surgeon
The University Hospital Southampton NHS Foundation Trust
The Wessex Cardiovascular and Thoracic Centre
Southampton General Hospital,
Southampton, United Kingdom

References

[1] Laennec RTH. Traité du diagnostic des maladies des poumons et du coeur. Tome Second. Paris: Brosson and Chaudé; 1819;(4)

[2] Ruckley CV, McCormack RJM. The management of spontaneous pneumothorax. Thorax. 1966;**21**:139-144

[3] Cerfolio RJ, Bryant AS. The management of chest tubes after pulmonary resection. Thoracic Surgery Clinics. 2010;**20**(3):399-405

Chapter 1

Indications of Surgery in Pneumothorax

Hany Hasan Elsayed

Abstract

Spontaneous pneumothorax (SP) is a type of collection of air in the pleural cavity that develops in the absence of trauma or iatrogenic cause. Its management has been a matter of debate for many decades. Nevertheless, clear guidelines from the American, British and European societies have been published. In this chapter, we will discuss the different society guidelines and the inter-guideline variations. We will also discuss the author's perspective for management of first-time pneumothorax which is an unsettled issue between respiratory physicians and thoracic surgeons. Finally, deviation from clinical guidelines is usually associated with deficient patient care, and in this chapter, the reflection on patient care from not following the pneumothorax guidelines will be discussed in detail.

Keywords: spontaneous pneumothorax, guidelines, first-time attack, indication for surgery, chest tube, primary pneumothorax, secondary pneumothorax

1. Introduction

Spontaneous pneumothorax (SP) is a type of collection of air in the pleural cavity that develops in the absence of trauma or iatrogenic cause [1, 2]. It is further classified as primary and secondary SP (PSP/SSP). While PSP affects patients with no clinically apparent lung disorders but small subpleural blebs/bullae, SSP involves an underlying pulmonary disease, which most often is chronic obstructive pulmonary disease (COPD) [2]. Spontaneous pneumothorax is a significant health burden, with annual incidences of 18–28 and 1.2–6 cases per 100,000 men and women, respectively [3]. The annual incidences of PSP among men and women are 7.4–18 (age-adjusted incidence) and 1.2–6 cases per 100,000 population, respectively; the annual incidences of SSP are similar, approximately 6.3 and 2 cases per 100,000 men and women, respectively [3].

Patients usually present with chest pain or breathlessness or both. Associated haemodynamic instability is an indication of a tension pneumothorax. The pathophysiology of PSP is a ruptured bleb or bullae which is usually located at the apex of the upper lobe or less frequently in the apical segment of the lower lobe. There is no known predisposing factor for its rupture and the resultant pneumothorax. SSP is caused more frequently by rupture of bullae in an underlying diseased lung, most commonly due to COPD/emphysema. It carries a significantly higher risk than PSP with mortality approaching 15% mainly due to associated patient comorbidities and low pulmonary reserve [4]. These differences between PSP and SSP are appreciated in guideline recommendations for management of spontaneous pneumothorax.

2. Percutaneous needle aspiration or chest tube drainage?

The evidence for needle aspiration NA as the initial treatment for spontaneous pneumothorax has been growing over the years. It is a simple, safe procedure and the learning curve for performing it is shorter than the classic chest tube drainage (CTD). It can also be performed in an out-patient setting, and if patients do require hospitalization, it usually requires a shorter hospital stay. Despite this, the guideline for using NA as an initial intervention is more evident in the European guidelines in comparison to the American guidelines for management of spontaneous pneumothorax.

The British Thoracic Society (BTS) guideline [5] and European Respiratory Society (ERS) task force statement [6] recommend aspiration as the first intervention, when needed, for all PSP without tension or haemodynamic instability. The BTS guideline is considered more modest for SSP: Needle aspiration can be considered for symptomatic patients with small spontaneous pneumothorax in an attempt to avoid CTD. On the other hand, the American College of Chest Physicians (ACCP) guideline [7] does not include needle aspiration for any patients with spontaneous pneumothorax. The classification of a small pneumothorax in the BTS guidelines is <2 cm on a chest X-ray.

Publication	No of patients	Includes SSP patients	Median hospital stay	Other outcomes	Recurrence rate
Harvey and Prescott, BMJ, 1994 [11]	73 (NA 35 and CTD 38)	No	3.2 vs. 5.3 (P = 0.005)	Total pain score was less with NA 2.7 vs. 6.7 (P < 0.001)	5/35 vs. 10/38 (P = 0.4)
Andrivet et al., Chest, 1995 [12]	61 (NA 33 and CTD 28)	Yes	7 vs. 7 days	CTD superior success 93% vs. 7% (P = 0.01)	29% NA vs. 14% CTD at 3 months (not significant)
Noppen et al., Am J Resp Crit Care Med, 2002 [13]	60 patients (NA 27 and CTD 33)	No	NA 54% vs. CTD 100% (P < 0.001)	1-week success rate NA 93% vs. CTD 85% (P = 0.4)	NA 26% vs. CTD 27.3% at 1 year (not significant)
Ayed et al., Eur Resp J, 2006 [14]	137 (NA 65 and CTD 72)	No	NA 1.8 days vs. CTD 4 days (P = 0.0003)	Immediate success in favour of CTD (68% vs. 62%, not significant), complications more with CTD	At 3 months NA 15% vs. CTD 8% (not significant)
Parlak et al., Resp Med, 2012 [15]	56 (NA 25 and CTD 31)	No	NA 2.4 vs. CTD 4.4 (P = 0.02)	Immediate success rate NA 60% vs. CTD 80.6% (P = 0.28)	At 1 year NA 4% vs. CTD 12.9% (P = 0.37)
Korczynski et al., Adv Exp Med Biol, 2015 [16]	49 (NA 22 and CTD 27)	No	NA 2 days vs. CTD 6 days (P < 0.05)	Immediate success rate NA 64% vs. CTD 82% (not significant)	Not measured

Table 1.
Studies comparing needle aspiration with chest tube drainage for management of spontaneous pneumothorax.

In cases of CTD, the BTS guidelines in 2003 [8] recommended insertion of the tube in the safety triangle of the chest to minimize the risks of possible injuries caused by the tube. The guidelines encourage physicians and surgeons to use the triangle in simple non-complicated pneumothoraces.

In a Cochrane review by Wakai et al. [9], they found no significant difference between simple needle aspiration and intercostal tube drainage for initial management of PSP regarding early failure rate, immediate success rate, duration of hospitalization, 1-year success rate and number of patients requiring pleurodesis at 1 year. Simple needle aspiration was associated with a reduction in the percentage of patients hospitalized when comparing it with intercostal tube insertion. Again, another recent meta-analysis by Kim and his colleagues [10] comparing seven studies for initial management of primary spontaneous pneumothorax showed that the recurrence rate of aspiration and intercostal tube drainage did not differ significantly, and again NA was associated with a shorter hospital patient stay. NA was however associated with inferior results regarding early resolution of pneumothorax in comparison to CTD. **Table 1** summarizes the studies performed showing the efficacy of NA in both PSP and SSP.

3. Indications of intervention according to the guidelines

The European Respiratory Society task force [6] for management of primary spontaneous pneumothorax has suggested five indications for definitive management: second-attack pneumothorax, persistent air leak 3–5 days, haemopneumothorax, bilateral pneumothorax and special occupations (divers and pilots).

The BTS guidelines [5, 8] agree with the same indications. The 2003 guidelines [8] had specified persistent air leak for 5 days in PSP and 3 days in SSP, but the 2010 [5] guidelines mention 5–7 days as an arbitrary number for persistent air leak for both PSP and SSP. The reason for giving a longer time period in PSP to wait for in the 2003 guidelines is that there is a better chance of healing of a ruptured bullae/bleb with the underlying normal lungs with PSP, while in SSP, the diseased lungs have a lower chance of sealing the leaking lesion if they have not done so in the first 3 days. The guidelines also add pregnancy as an indication for intervention.

The ACCP guidelines [7] mention 4 days of conservative treatment in patients with persistent air leak after drain insertion for spontaneous pneumothorax before surgical intervention. Again, the same indications mentioned by other guidelines are considered in the Delphi consensus statement.

The main indication in all guidelines for definitive intervention in cases of PSP and SSP is recurrence. The reason behind this is that the chances of a pneumothorax not recurring after the first attack are usually more than the chances recurring, and hence patients after the first attack are given a chance of no intervention provided their first pneumothorax has healed. Chances of recurrence after a second attack (ipsilateral or contralateral) are in the range of 60–80%, and hence patients are not usually offered the conservative option. Opponents of this opinion would argue that the chances of recurrence after the first attack are still too high to be acceptable for any logical patient. Estimates of the incidence of recurrent PSP range from 25 to more than 50%, with most recurrences seen within the first year [17]. As an example, a study of 153 patients with PSP found a recurrence rate of 54% [18].

Female gender, tall stature in men, low body weight and failure to stop smoking have been associated with an increased risk of recurrence [18, 19]. Unfortunately, most patients have a very unpleasant experience with their first attack of pneumothorax. The sensation of chest pain with breathlessness sounds like 'I felt I am going to die' as patients may express. The other unpleasant experience is insertion of a

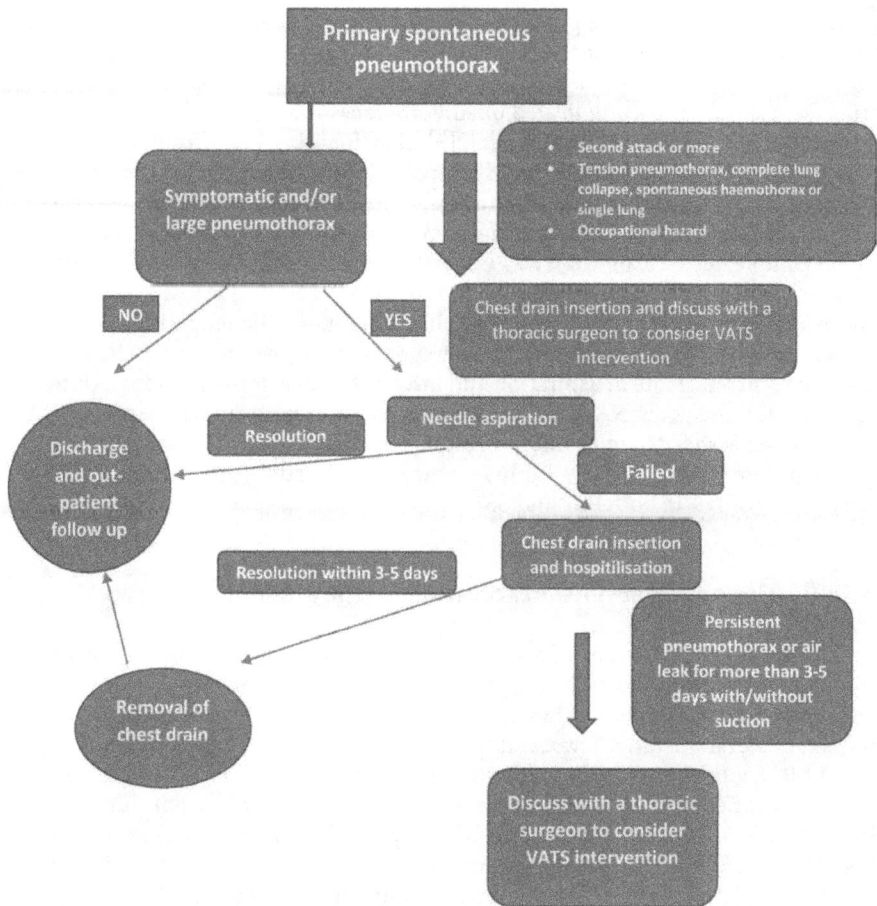

Figure 1.
Simple flowchart summary for management of primary spontaneous pneumothorax.

chest drain for drainage which is very frequently painful even with using generous local anaesthesia. These experiences usually form a painful memory scar for the patients and their parents which they would not like to experience again if the intervention to treat it carries a very low risk.

Figure 1 shows a flowchart summary recommended by the author for the different published guidelines for indications of intervention in primary spontaneous pneumothorax.

4. Guidelines for management of first-attack pneumothorax

In recent years there has been a trend towards a more conservative approach to management of primary spontaneous pneumothorax, based on the principle that intrapleural air does not necessarily require a therapeutic intervention and that management depends on the clinical symptoms and not on the size of the pneumothorax [20]. This conservative approach may be appropriate as tension pneumothorax from a PSP is extremely rare [21]. In selected patients with minimal or no symptoms and good access to medical care in case of deterioration, observation alone may be appropriate.

Within the current British Thoracic Society guidelines (from 2010), there is a significant emphasis on a conservative approach to treatment [5] with management predominantly based on clinical symptoms. In contrast, the American College of Chest Physicians Delphi consensus statement (from 2001) recommended a more aggressive approach, with intercostal drain placement recommended in any pneumothorax larger than 20% of the hemithorax, irrespective of the symptoms [7].

Patients with an attack of tension pneumothorax (quite rare in PSP) and more commonly patients with a first attack associated with complete lung collapse should be counselled about the benefits of definitive intervention with VATS due to the life-threatening condition of a tension pneumothorax or the higher than usual risk of recurrence associated with a complete collapsed lung. This is probably due to an associated larger bulla with a completely collapsed lung, and hence the chances of re rupture seem higher than a simple smaller size pneumothorax attack which is usually associated with a bleb or small bulla.

It is in the previous context that current clinical practice guidelines for management of spontaneous pneumothorax tend to avoid use of surgery for patients with only a single episode of PSP. The trauma—considering not only physical but also perhaps psychological—of receiving such major surgery for a simple benign disease in a young patient was considered quite excessive if the recurrence rate of attacks is not high. The 2003 British Thoracic Surgery Guidelines for the management of spontaneous pneumothorax specifically referred to an open thoracotomy as the 'gold standard' for surgical management [8].

With this in mind, it would be unsurprising that clinicians are reluctant to offer such aggressive surgery. This is reflected in those guidelines listing the indications for surgery to only be first contralateral pneumothorax, second ipsilateral pneumothorax, synchronous bilateral spontaneous pneumothorax, single attack of tension pneumothorax, a persistent air leak after chest drain insertion, and spontaneous significant haemothorax [5–8]. First episode PSP is deliberately excluded. In a similar context back in 2001, the American College of Chest Physicians consensus statement on the management of spontaneous pneumothorax explicitly states that 'procedures to prevent the recurrence of a primary spontaneous pneumothorax should be reserved for the second pneumothorax occurrence' [7].

It is therefore evident that views on surgical indications are influenced by the perceived harm from surgery, the aggression of intervention and the simplicity of the disease. Over the past decade or more since the above guidelines, the trauma from thoracotomy remains existing. What we think has changed, though, is the current view of whether an open thoracotomy remains the surgical approach of choice across the world.

The combination of lowered morbidity with equivalent efficacy at preventing recurrence means that open thoracotomy should no longer be regarded as the first-line approach for the surgical management of PSP [22, 23]. Today, VATS has become the approach of choice by surgeons throughout the world, and it is rare to find traumatic open thoracotomy being offered to young patients with PSP especially that many are young patients and could be manual workers where thoracotomy would be an obstacle to perform their job satisfactorily. Compared to the 2003 version, the latest British Thoracic Surgery Guidelines for the management of spontaneous pneumothorax published in 2010 pointedly no longer uses the words 'gold standard' in relation to open thoracotomy [5, 8]. Instead, it is very noticeable that when the latest guidelines advised surgical pleurodesis for specific circumstances (such as pregnancy), VATS is the only approach named, and open thoracotomy is nowhere to be seen.

In summary, the management of a first-attack pneumothorax according to the current guidelines is debatable and incoherent. Advice will range from conservative

Ref.	No. of patients	Chest drain duration	Length of stay	Follow-up	Recurrence	Cost	Other
Schramel et al., ERJ [24]	149 first episode PSP VATS: 70 Chest drain: 79	(Both first and recurrent episode included)	(Both first and recurrent episode included)	Chest drain: 96 ± 18 months VATS: 29 ± 10 months	1 year: VATS (3%) < CD (19%) 2 years: VATS (4%) < CD (22%)	VATS < chest drain cost of treating recurrence: VATS similar to chest drain	
Torresini et al., EJCTS [25]	70 chest drain: 35 VATS: 35	VATS: 3.9 days Chest drain: 9 days	VATS: 6 days Chest drain: 12 days	12 months	VATS: 2.8% Chest drain: 22.8%	VATS: $1925 Chest drain: $2750 (cost of recurrence also included)	Secondary pneumothorax included chest drain arm: 2 VATS arm: 4
Chou et al., ICTVS [26]	VATS: 51	2 days (54%)	3 days (54%)	38 months	0	—	
Margolis et al., ATS [27]	VATS: 156	—	2.4 ± 0.5 days	2–96 months (median: 62 months)	0	—	Talc poudrage for all patients intra-op
Sawada et al., Chest [28]	281 Chest drain: 181 Thoracotomy: 13 VATS: 87	—	Chest drain: 14.5 days Thoracotomy: 22.2 days VATS: 8.3 days (P < 0.001)	13–163 months (mean: 78.3 months) Not specified for first episode cases	Chest drain: 54.7% Thoracotomy: 7.7% VATS: 10.3% (P < 0.001) (thoracotomy vs. VATS: P = 0.61)		Length of stay analysis included both first and recurrent episodes
Chen et al., ATS [29]	52 chest drain 22 VATS: 30	—	VATS: 4.8 Chest drain: 6.1 (P = 0.034)	3–38 months (mean 16 months)	VATS: 3.3% Chest drain: 22.7% (P = 0.038)	Total cost of 1 hospital stay VATS: $1273 Chest drain: $865	All patients had failed initial needle aspiration

Table 2.
Studies using video-assisted thoracoscopy for management of first-attack spontaneous pneumothorax.

management of 'doing nothing' up to a VATS intervention on the next available list. Needle aspiration and chest tube drainage are commonly used modalities, but CTD will remain the most common and classic intervention for an attack of pneumothorax worldwide. It is the author's preference to send patients for a VATS intervention on the next available list without inserting a chest tube (provided there is no respiratory compromise) to allow a shorter hospital stay, allow patients to return to work or school as early as possible and most importantly avoid the high risk of recurrence. **Table 2** shows studies starting more than two decades ago considering VATS for first-attack pneumothorax.

A conservative approach with follow-up or needle aspiration seems as a reasonable first-line option in a first-attack small-sized pneumothorax. In patients with a large pneumothorax who are not keen for surgery or with hospital logistics that would hinder the availability of VATS intervention on the next morning list due to lack of facilities or personnel, a chest drain insertion is the most reasonable option. Further intervention will then be guided by the time of resolution of the pneumothorax, availability of a VATS intervention service and patient wishes after understanding the risks of recurrence after the first attack.

5. Guideline recommendations for lifestyle changes post pneumothorax

Recommendations for passengers travelling by air after an attack of pneumothorax was largely based on anecdotal case reports [30, 31]. A pneumothorax, especially an undrained one, is however an absolute contraindication to all commercial air travels [32]. Travelling with a chest drain inserted for pneumothorax had no published guidelines or recommendations. It is theoretically safe, but most airlines would not be willing to accept such a risk and would need documented medical input and insurance approval to allow patients to travel.

According to the BTS guidelines, commercial airlines advise individuals to avoid air travel for 6 weeks after an episode of primary spontaneous pneumothorax and stress that patients should not fly until resolution has been confirmed [8].

Although there is no evidence that recurrence is caused by flying, the consequences of a pneumothorax occurring during a flight could be serious because of the lack of medical care. Restrictions on flying may be more justified in patients for whom pneumothorax is associated with higher risk, such as smokers and patients with underlying lung disease (secondary spontaneous pneumothorax). In patients with secondary pneumothorax who have not been treated surgically, air travel should be avoided for 1 year after an episode (grade C recommendation). Patients with a history of pneumothorax who have not been treated surgically should also be advised against practising high-risk sports, such as diving (grade C recommendation) [8].

The performance of a VATS procedure can offer patients more safety to fly or practise diving sports. This makes patients with occupations as pilots and scuba divers candidates for a VATS intervention even with a first-attack pneumothorax. Definitive treatment significantly reduces the risk of recurrence and makes air travel safer from an airline point of view [30]; however, an individual clinical decision is usually made by the treating clinician, considering both airline policy and details of relevant insurance.

There are no specific guidelines regarding lifestyle modification to prevent patients from having another attack of pneumothorax apart from advising all patients to stop smoking. Despite the apparent relationship between smoking and pneumothorax, 80–86% of young patients continue to smoke after their first episode of PSP [33]. Smoking cessation remains the only reversible risk factor known to reduce the chance of recurrence although we should not neglect the deleterious role of marijuana and cannabis smoking as a risk of PSP. From the author's point of view, cannabis has a more destructive effect on the lung parenchyma exposing patients to a higher risk of first-attack and recurrent pneumothorax. This has also been noted elsewhere [34]. Smoking cessation advice is therefore given to all our patients who smoke after the first episode of spontaneous pneumothorax.

6. Hazards of non-compliance with pneumothorax guidelines

Despite the availability of published guidelines, there has been a recording in the English literature of non-compliance or deviation from the guidelines, which has occasionally resulted in inconsistency or patient harm in management of spontaneous pneumothorax. We have previously published our experience in a large UK tertiary centre [35] where the median time to referral from chest physicians to thoracic surgeons after the 2003 BTS guideline publication was 10 days for a persistent pneumothorax which is longer than any time suggested by all guidelines. This has resulted in a higher incidence of developing empyema and the more frequent need of a thoracotomy rather than VATS treatment for patients with delayed referral. Delayed referral is one of the most common areas of deviation from published pneumothorax guidelines.

When assessing a pneumothorax, the size will determine the initial step of management, ranging from conservative treatment, needle aspiration up to chest tube drainage in larger pneumothoraces. There is discrepancy in size calculations of pneumothorax between different guidelines, and this has resulted in inconsistency in management. Kelly and Clooney have noticed this with management of 234 patients managed in Australia [36], and patients with a large pneumothorax were treated conservatively. Yoon et al. have studied size calculation of PSP in 87 patients in a tertiary UK centre and found significant discrepancy between the size calculation suggested in the BTS guidelines (resulting in only 70% compliance) and the ACCP guidelines (resulting in only 32% compliance) with consequent inconsistent management [37]. Sole blame on physicians and surgeons applying the guidelines can be unfair as there is obvious inconsistency in size calculation between different pneumothorax guidelines [38], and estimation of the size using only a chest X-ray can yield variable results [39].

The BTS guidelines [8] suggest explicitly inserting a chest drain for simple spontaneous pneumothorax in the 'safe triangle of chest'. We have previously published that knowledge of the guidelines regarding this site of insertion is deficient in surgeons and physicians involved in insertion of chest drains [40]. This resulted in more than 50% of drains inserted being outside the 'safe triangle' exposing patients to an unnecessary risk of higher morbidity associated with this common everyday procedure.

7. Summary

To conclude, the current guidelines available for treatment of spontaneous pneumothorax would state that in cases of spontaneous pneumothorax, patients will be assessed for clinical status and size of pneumothorax. In a very small PSP pneumothorax with no clinical complaint, it would be reasonable to discharge the patient and follow up. All patients with SSP require hospital admission. In a sizable pneumothorax with symptoms, the BTS and ERS guidelines would recommend needle aspiration with chest drain insertion if failed. The ACCP guidelines would recommend a chest drain straightaway. If the pneumothorax persists for 3–7 days according to different guidelines, definitive treatment is required. The BTS, ACCP and ERS guidelines choose first-attack tension pneumothorax, bilateral pneumothoraces and special occupations (pilots and divers) as indications for definitive intervention after one attack of spontaneous pneumothorax, while the BTS guidelines add pregnancy and previous pneumonectomy as indications.

All guidelines agree that second-attack ipsilateral and first-attack contralateral recurrent pneumothorax are indications for intervention. The management of first-attack pneumothorax is debatable in all guidelines and will range from conservative management up to performing a VATS for definitive treatment. This will depend on the clinical situation, availability of resources/personnel and patient wishing to avoid the relatively high chance of recurrence. With the advancement in VATS techniques and significant reduction in risk of recurrence with a VATS intervention, it could be reasonable to perform the procedure on the next available list. A VATS procedure should be the standard surgical procedure for pneumothorax patients, and an open thoracotomy is no longer considered the 'gold standard' in all guidelines. All patients with an attack of spontaneous pneumothorax need lifestyle modifications regarding their smoking status, sport activity and travelling through air flights.

Physicians and thoracic surgeons should be aware of the current available guidelines for management of spontaneous pneumothorax. Deviation from the guidelines, particularly regarding the time to refer patients for definitive treatment, is associated with higher patient morbidity (particularly developing an empyema), increased hospital stay and higher medical costs.

Author details

Hany Hasan Elsayed
Thoracic Surgery, Ain Shams University, Cairo, Egypt

*Address all correspondence to: drhany.elsayed@yahoo.co.uk

IntechOpen

References

[1] Noppen M, De Keukeleire T. Pneumothorax. Respiration. 2008;**76**(2):121-127

[2] Gupta D, Hansell A, Nichols T, Duong T, Ayres JG, Strachan D. Epidemiology of pneumothorax in England. Thorax. 2000;**55**(8):666-671

[3] Noppen M. Spontaneous pneumothorax: Epidemiology, pathophysiology and cause. European Respiratory Review. 2010;**19**(117):217-219

[4] Won Choi II. Pneumothorax. Tuberculosis Respiratory Disease. 2014;**76**(3):99-104

[5] MacDuff A, Arnold A, Harvey J. Management of spontaneous pneumothorax: British Thoracic Society Pleural Disease Guideline 2010. Thorax. 2010;**65**(Suppl 2):ii18-ii31

[6] Tschopp JM, Bintcliffe O, Astoul P, Canalis E, Driesen P, Janssen J, et al. ERS task force statement: Diagnosis and treatment of primary spontaneous pneumothorax. The European Respiratory Journal. 2015;**46**(2):321-335

[7] Baumann MH, Strange C, Heffner JE, Light R, Kirby TJ, Klein J, et al. Management of spontaneous pneumothorax: An American College of Chest Physicians Delphi consensus statement. Chest. 2001;**119**:590-602

[8] Henry M, Arnold T, Harvey J. BTS guidelines for the management of spontaneous pneumothorax. Thorax. 2003;**58**(Suppl 2):ii39-ii52

[9] Wakai A, O'Sullivan RG, McCabe G. Simple aspiration versus intercostal tube drainage for primary spontaneous pneumothorax in adults. Cochrane Database of Systematic Reviews. 2007;**1**:CD004479

[10] Kim MJ, Park I, Park JM, et al. Systematic review and meta-analysis of initial management of pneumothorax in adults: Intercostal tube drainage versus other invasive methods. PLoS ONE. 2017;**12**:e0178802

[11] Harvey J, Prescott RJ. Simple aspiration versus intercostal tube drainage for spontaneous pneumothorax in patients with normal lungs. British Thoracic Society Research Committee. BMJ. 1994;**309**:1338-1339

[12] Andrivet P, Djedaini K, Teboul JL, et al. Spontaneous pneumothorax. Comparison of thoracic drainage vs immediate or delayed needle aspiration. Chest. 1995;**108**:335-339

[13] Noppen M, Alexander P, Driesen P, et al. Manual aspiration versus chest tube drainage in first episodes of primary spontaneous pneumothorax: A multicenter, prospective, randomized pilot study. American Journal of Respiratory and Critical Care Medicine. 2002;**165**:1240-1244

[14] Ayed AK, Chandrasekaran C, Sukumar M. Aspiration versus tube drainage in primary spontaneous pneumothorax: A randomised study. The European Respiratory Journal. 2006;**27**:477-482

[15] Parlak M, Uil SM, van den Berg JW. A prospective, randomised trial of pneumothorax therapy: Manual aspiration versus conventional chest tube drainage. Respiratory Medicine. 2012;**106**:1600-1605

[16] Korczyński P, Górska K, Nasiłowski J, et al. Comparison of small bore catheter aspiration and chest tube drainage in the management of spontaneous pneumothorax. Advances in Experimental Medicine and Biology. 2015;**866**:15-23

[17] Light RW. Pleural Diseases. 6th ed. Philadelphia: Lippincott, Williams and Wilkins; 2013

[18] Sadikot RT, Greene T, Meadows K, Arnold AG. Recurrence of primary spontaneous pneumothorax. Thorax. 1997;**52**:805

[19] Guo Y, Xie C, Rodriguez RM, Light RW. Factors related to recurrence of spontaneous pneumothorax. Respirology. 2005;**10**:378

[20] Hsu HH, Chen JS. The etiology and therapy of primary spontaneous pneumothoraces. Expert Review of Respiratory Medicine. 2015;**9**(5):655-665

[21] Roberts DJ, Leigh-Smith S, Faris PD, Blackmore C, Ball CG, Robertson HL, et al. Clinical presentation of patients with tension pneumothorax: A systematic review. Annals of Surgery. 2015;**261**(6):1068-1078

[22] Dagnegård HH, Rosén A, Sartipy U, Bergman P. Recurrence rate after thoracoscopic surgery for primary spontaneous pneumothorax. Scandinavian Cardiovascular Journal. 2017;**51**(4):228-232

[23] Joshi V, Kirmani B, Zacharias J. Thoracotomy versus VATS: Is there an optimal approach to treating pneumothorax? Annals of the Royal College of Surgeons of England. 2013;**95**(1):61-64

[24] Schramel FM, Sutedja TG, Braber JC, van Mourik JC, Postmus PE. Cost-effectiveness of video-assisted thoracoscopic surgery versus conservative treatment for first time or recurrent spontaneous pneumothorax. The European Respiratory Journal. 1996;**9**:1821-1825

[25] Torresini G, Vaccarili M, Divisi D, Crisci R. Is video-assisted thoracic surgery justified at first spontaneous pneumothorax? European Journal of Cardio-Thoracic Surgery. 2001;**20**:42-45

[26] Chou SH, Cheng YJ, Kao EL. Is video-assisted thoracic surgery indicated in the first episode primary spontaneous pneumothorax? Interactive Cardiovascular and Thoracic Surgery. 2003;**2**:552-554

[27] Margolis M, Gharagozloo F, Tempesta B, Trachiotis GD, Katz NM, Alexander EP. Video-assisted thoracic surgical treatment of initial spontaneous pneumothorax in young patients. The Annals of Thoracic Surgery. 2003;**76**:1661-1663

[28] Sawada S, Watanabe Y, Moriyama S. Video-assisted thoracoscopic surgery for primary spontaneous pneumothorax: Evaluation of indications and long-term outcome compared with conservative treatment and open thoracotomy. Chest. 2005;**127**:2226-2230

[29] Chen JS, Hsu HH, Tsai KT, Yuan A, Chen WJ, Lee YC. Salvage for unsuccessful aspiration of primary pneumothorax: Thoracoscopic surgery or chest tube drainage? The Annals of Thoracic Surgery. 2008;**85**:1908-1913

[30] Ahmedzai S, Balfour-Lynn IM, Bewick T, et al. Managing passengers with stable respiratory disease planning air travel: British thoracic society recommendations. Thorax. 2011;**66**(Suppl. 1):i1-i30

[31] Hu X, Cowl CT, Baqir M, et al. Air travel and pneumothorax. Chest. 2014;**145**:688-694

[32] Duchateau FX, Legrand JM, Verner L, et al. Commercial aircraft repatriation of patients with pneumothorax. Air Medical Journal. 2013;**32**:200-202

[33] Smit HJM, Chatrou M, Postmus PE. The impact of spontaneous pneumothorax, and its treatment, on the smoking behaviour of young

adult smokers. Respiratory Medicine. 1998;**92**:1132-1136

[34] Hedevang Olesen W, Katballe N, Sindby JE, Titlestad IL, Andersen PE, Ekholm O, et al. Cannabis increased the risk of primary spontaneous pneumothorax in tobacco smokers: A case-control study. European Journal of Cardio-Thoracic Surgery. 2017;**52**(4):679-685

[35] Elsayed H, Kent W, McShane J, Page R, Shackcloth M. Treatment of pneumothoraces at a tertiary Centre: Are we following the current guidelines? Interactive Cardiovascular and Thoracic Surgery. 2011;**12**(3):430-433

[36] Kelly AM, Clooney M. Deviation from published guidelines in the management of primary spontaneous pneumothorax in Australia. Internal Medicine Journal. 2008;**38**(1):64-67

[37] Yoon J, Sivakumar P, O'Kane K, Ahmed L. A need to reconsider guidelines on management of primary spontaneous pneumothorax? International Journal of Emergency Medicine. 2017;**10**:9

[38] Kelly AM, Drudy D. Comparison of size classification of primary spontaneous pneumothorax by three international guidelines: A case for international consensus? Respiratory Medicine. 2008;**102**(12):1830-1832

[39] Salazar AJ, Aguirre DA, Ocampo J, Camacho JC, Díaz XA. Evaluation of three pneumothorax size quantification methods on digitized chest X-ray films using medical-grade grayscale and consumer-grade color displays. Journal of Digital Imaging. 2014;**27**(2):280-286

[40] Elsayed H, Roberts R, Emadi M, Whittle I, Shackcloth M. Chest drain insertion is not a harmless procedure: Are we doing it safely? Interactive Cardiovascular and Thoracic Surgery. 2010;**11**(6):745-748

Chapter 2

Primary Spontaneous Pneumothorax, a Clinical Challenge

Fabian Andres Giraldo Vallejo, Rubby Romero, Melissa Mejia and Estefania Quijano

Abstract

Primary spontaneous pneumothorax (PSP) is a common disease in medical practice that affects young healthy people with a significant recurrence rate. PSP is the presence of air in the pleural space not caused by injury or medical intervention. Some risk factors include male gender, age, and smoking. Classic clinical presentation starts with acute-onset chest pain and shortness of breath. Physical examination can be normal in small pneumothoraces, but in larger pneumothoraces, breath sounds and tactile fremitus are typically decreased or absent, and percussion is hyperresonant. Chest X-ray can help confirm the diagnosis. Evacuation of air from the pleural cavity and prevention of future recurrences are the primary goals of treatment and depend on the patient's presentation. Initial deciding factors to direct the management are first-time or recurrent spontaneous pneumothorax and size of the pneumothorax. Treatment may include conventional chest tube drainage, video-assisted thoracoscopic surgery (VATS), or open surgery.

Keywords: pneumothorax, pleural cavity, chest tube drainage, video-assisted thoracoscopic surgery

1. Introduction

Pneumothorax is defined as an abnormal collection of air in the pleural cavity, which is a potential space between the two pleurae (visceral and parietal) of the lungs [1]. Itard, a student of Laennec, first coined pneumothorax in 1803, but it was not until 1932 that it was realized that spontaneous pneumothorax was not always caused by tuberculosis. Pneumothorax is classified as spontaneous, traumatic, or iatrogenic (**Figure 1**). Primary spontaneous pneumothorax (PSP) occurs in patients without underlying lung disease or without a precipitating event, and it is a common disease in medical practice with a significant global health problem affecting adolescent and young adults. Notwithstanding the absence of pulmonary disease, many of these patients have asymptomatic subpleural blebs and bullae; they are found in up to 90% of cases at thoracoscopy or thoracotomy and in up to 80% of cases on CT scanning of the thorax [2]. PSP is a benign condition, which resolves spontaneously in the majority of cases [3]. Secondary spontaneous pneumothorax is a complication of a preexisting lung disease and the major causes in descending order are airway disease (chronic obstructive pulmonary disease or cystic fibrosis),

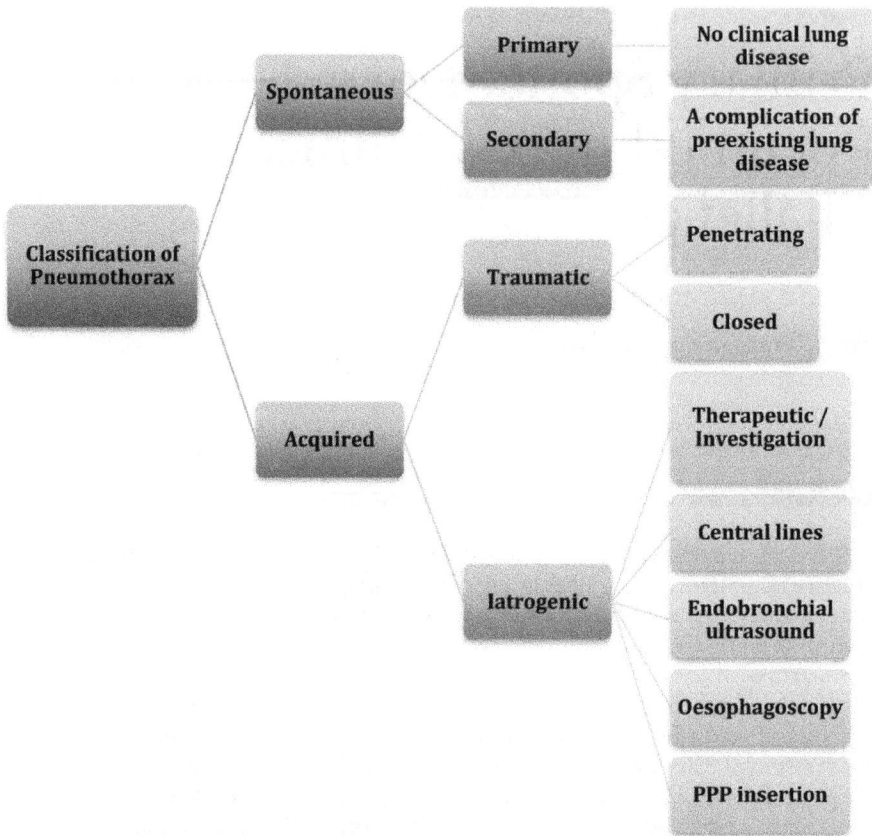

Figure 1.
*Classification of pneumothorax. Adapted from Noppen M. European Respiratory Review. 2010;**19**:217–219.*

infectious lung disease, interstitial lung disease (sarcoidosis), connective tissue disease (Marfan syndrome or Ehlers-Danlos syndrome), cancer, and thoracic endometriosis. Traumatic pneumothorax is caused by penetrating and non-penetrating (blunt) trauma to the chest. Iatrogenic pneumothorax results from a complication of a diagnostic or therapeutic intervention [4].

The most important risk factor of primary spontaneous pneumothorax is tobacco smoking, and the number of cigarettes smoked per day contributes to the increased risk. Cannabis smoking is associated with bullous disease. Smoking suspension is the only modifiable risk factor for recurrence of PSP. Catamenial pneumothorax is a rare condition associated with the presence of thoracic endometriosis and affects women before or after 72 hours of the start of menstruation. Other risks include male gender and age with peaking between 15 and 34 years. Clinical presentation in patients with spontaneous pneumothorax depends on the size of pneumothorax. PSP may be asymptomatic or may be suspected by typical clinical features. The most common symptoms are abrupt onset of chest pain and breathlessness; the findings on physical exam may include absent breath sounds, reduced ipsilateral chest expansion, and hyperresonant percussion [5]. The presence of hypotension and tachycardia may indicate tension pneumothorax that occurs when the intrapleural pressure exceeded atmospheric pressure, caused mediastinal deviation, and reduced venous return and cardiovascular collapse [6]. The diagnosis is suggested by patient's history and findings on examination and is confirmed with chest X-ray;

the radiographic sign is the displacement of the pleural line and an absence of lung markings between the edge of the pleura and chest wall. Computed tomography (CT) provides sensitive and specific imaging for the detection of pneumothorax, but it is not recommended routinely except if loculated pneumothorax or lung disease is suspected. The diagnosis may be clearly made on a chest radiograph, and an excess radiation dose should be avoided in this young patient population [7].

The difference between primary, secondary, traumatic, and iatrogenic pneumothorax is important to be defined because of the different management strategies required for their treatment. The goal of treatment is to remove the air from the pleural space and decrease the recurrence. Management options range from observation to aspiration or drainage to thoracic surgical intervention and is guided by presenting symptoms: hemodynamic compromise, size and cause of pneumothorax. As well as it is the first time or recurring pneumothorax. PSP can be treated conservatively; patients with first episode who are asymptomatic and have a small pneumothorax need simple clinical observation, analgesia, and oxygen therapy that increased the rate of reabsorption. The removal of air from the pleural space can be achieved with needle aspiration or chest drain insertion [7, 8]. Simple aspiration and chest tube drainage are the most frequently used methods for the initial treatment of primary spontaneous pneumothorax. Aspiration should be the primary treatment in uncomplicated cases; the insertion of an aspiration catheter is easier and safer than chest tube drainage and is recommended in the guidelines. Chest tube drainage is the most popular and recommended air evacuation technique, but this method does not provide any definitive recurrence prevention [9, 10]. Video-assisted thoracic surgery (VATS) is a minimally invasive procedure, and its advantages include less postoperative pain, better postoperative pulmonary function, shorter length of hospital stay, and less invasive than thoracotomy. Thoracoscopic evaluation of primary pneumothorax shows that this disorder is regularly associated with apical subpleural blebs or bullae. Pleurodesis, either mechanical or chemical, using talc has to be applied to decrease the risk of recurrence of PSP [11, 12]. Open thoracotomy plus pleurectomy are used in the case of recurrent ipsilateral PSP, simultaneous bilateral PSP, an episode of PSP following a previous episode of contralateral PSP, first episode of tension pneumothorax, significant spontaneous hemopneumothorax at first episode, persistent air leak through the chest tube for more than 5–7 days, or failure of the lung to reexpand despite adequate pleural space drainage in the first episode. Open surgery has the lower recurrence rate [13]. The main complication of primary spontaneous pneumothorax is recurrence, which is greater after conservative treatment. Some risk factors for recurrence are younger age, male sex, and low body mass index [14]. A preventive procedure like thoracotomy or thoracoscopy plus pleurodesis may be recommended after the first episode of pneumothorax, with the objective to reduce the rate of recurrence. Some agents have been investigated for pleurodesis, but talc poudrage has presented the best results until now [15].

2. Epidemiology

Pneumothorax is defined as the presence of air in the pleural space. For air to enter into the pleural space from the capillary blood would require pleural pressure lower than -54 mmHg (< -36 cm H_2O), which is difficult to obtain in normal circumstances [16].

If air is present in the pleural space, some of these events may have occurred:

1. Communication between alveola and pleura

2. Communication between the atmosphere (direct or indirect) and the pleural space

3. Presence of gas-producing organisms in the pleural space

PSP has an incidence of 7.4 to 18 cases per 100,000 population each year in males and 1.2 to 6 cases per 100,000 populations each year in females [17, 18]. Risk factors for PSP include tall thin people, male sex, and smoking. The recurrence range is 25–50%, and most recurrences occur in the first year [19]. Female gender, tall male, low body weight, and persistent smoking are associated with a high rate of recurrence [20]. In the largest epidemiologic study of PSP from Bobbio et al. with 42,595 patients, they found that the mean age was significantly greater in women than in men (41 ± 19 vs. 37 ± 19 p < 0.0001), rehospitalization was more frequent in women than in men in patients aged <50 years (p < 0.0001). In the 50–64 years age group, surgical procedures and rehospitalizations were more frequent in men than in women (p = 0.002 and p < 0.0001, respectively). The most commonly performed procedures were thoracoscopic resection of blebs (52% of cases) and talc pleurodesis (24% of cases). Surgery was associated with younger age, secondary pneumothorax, and ICU surveillance (p < 0.001) [21]. Moderate smoking (22 cigarettes/day) increases the risk of first episode of PSP up to 22 times. PSP usually occurs at rest, so the lack of physical activity should be avoided in the counseling of these patients [17]. Thoracic endometriosis may lead to catamenial pneumothorax and should be considered in women with PSP temporally related to menstruation [22]. Malnutrition in patients with anorexia nervosa may lead to the development of PSP. Birt-Hogg-Dubé syndrome (which predisposes patients to benign skin tumors and renal cancers) is an autosomal dominant condition defined as a rare cause of PSP [23]. Precipitating factors include atmospheric pressure changes and exposure to loud music [24, 25].

An increased frequency of PSP is seen in patients with Marfan syndrome and homocystinuria. Marfan syndrome is a common inherited connective tissue disorder with typical skeletal, ocular, and cardiovascular manifestations. Pulmonary involvement occurs less frequently, with PSP being the most frequently reported. Karpman et al.'s study in 2011 found a prevalence of pneumothorax in patients with Marfan syndrome between and 11%. The increased risk of pneumothorax has been attributed to the presence of apical blebs, bullae, and abnormal connective tissue constituents in the lung parenchyma or increased mechanical stresses in the lung apices due to the tall body habitus. Patients who have Marfanoid features such as long stature, hyperextendable joints, and dislocated lens should be studied by CT scanning to identify blebs and bullae. This may allow risk stratification for pneumothorax in patients with this syndrome and also favors identification of aortic root disease, which leads to aneurysmal dilation, aortic regurgitation, and dissection [26, 27]. A multidisciplinary approach is fundamental in these patients and their family, who must be thoroughly investigated, to confirm the disease and to initiate the treatment, thus decreasing mortality, especially due to cardiovascular causes; also a medical genetics consultation should be provided for genetic counseling [28].

PSP recurrence rates are typically cited as between 16 and 52%, which makes counseling about future risk difficult and creates uncertainty regarding the optimal management. Thoracic Society guidelines advise that pneumothorax recurrence is an indication for surgery (whether second ipsilateral or first contralateral) [29]. Unfortunately, there is no consensus on which treatment offers the best reduction in risk of recurrence [6]. A systematic review demonstrates a 32% PSP recurrence rate, with almost all the risk in the first year. Recurrence rates did not differ based on the initial intervention for PSP. Female sex was associated with higher risk, suggesting possible sex-specific pathophysiology. Also lower BMI and radiological evidence of dystrophic lungs were associated with higher risk of recurrence (bullae on computed tomography (CT) and pleural thickening on chest radiography), until smoking cessation was associated with a fourfold decrease in risk [30].

3. Clinical presentation

Symptoms in primary spontaneous pneumothorax may be minimal or absent. These clinical symptoms depend on proportion and the size of the pneumothorax. Patients may present an abrupt onset of pleuritic chest pain associated with dyspnea and shortness of breath, and some patients may experience shoulder tip pain [29]. Severe symptoms are not common, and when this happens it suggests a tension pneumothorax. Typical examination findings in primary spontaneous pneumothorax include ipsilateral decreased breath sounds on auscultation, percussion hyperresonance, and thoracic hypoexpansion. The presence of observable breathlessness has influenced subsequent management in previous guidelines [29, 31]. Hemodynamic compromise is unusual in PSP. Arterial blood gas measurements are frequently abnormal in patients with pneumothorax. Arterial oxygen tension is lower according to the extent of the pneumothorax but oxygen saturations are adequate, and pulmonary function tests are poor predictors of the presence or size of a pneumothorax [32].

The clinical features in tension pneumothorax are shortness of breath, dyspnea, tachypnea, respiratory distress, hypoxemia, hypotension, tachycardia and ipsilateral decreased air entry, and percussion hyperresonance. This condition requires an urgent thoracic decompression when the diagnosis is suspected, and the clinicians should be prepared to perform urgent thoracic decompression without chest radiographic confirmation in these patients [31].

4. Diagnosis

4.1 Plain chest X-ray

The diagnosis of pneumothorax is usually confirmed by imaging techniques such as PA chest radiograph, and the excess radiation dose should be avoided in this young patient population. The diagnostic hallmark is the displacement of the pleural line. The pneumothorax is most frequently seen at the lung apex, but lateral, subpulmonic, and medial collections of air can also be seen [33]. Chest X-ray is the first diagnostic evaluation imaging being used, but small-sized pneumothoraces or loculated pneumothoraces can be missed on chest X-ray. If a pneumothorax is suspected and is unrevealed on chest X-ray, a more specific diagnostic imaging like chest computed tomography (CT) is necessary [34].

4.2 Ultrasonography

Ultrasound is a sensitive technique in the evaluation of respiratory diseases and was first used to diagnose pneumothorax in humans in 1987. Ultrasound is commonly used in emergency department with trauma patients and show significantly higher and quicker diagnostic accuracy than chest radiographs in these patients [35]. The routine use of ultrasound in PSP is not established.

4.3 CT and its indications

CT scanning is recommended for uncertain or complex cases and is useful in the detection of small pneumothoraces and size estimation. Emphysema, bullous lung, and another lung pathology are identified [29]. Chest CT is helpful in understanding the extent of the underlying lung parenchyma distraction. Some patients presented a loculated pneumothorax or pulmonary air cysts [34].

4.4 Size of pneumothorax

The clinical manifestations and evaluation are more important than the size of pneumothorax and do not correlate with the proportion of the pneumothorax [29]. The size of a pneumothorax is classified into three groups:

- Small is defined as small rim of air around the lung.

- Moderate is defined as collapsed halfway toward the heart border.

- Complete is defined as airless lung, separate from the diaphragm [2].

The difference of a small or large pneumothorax depends on the presence of visible rim <2 cm between the lung margin and the chest wall [29]. PA chest X-ray has been used to quantify the size of the pneumothorax. A commonly used method for estimating pneumothorax size is the light index. This method assumes that the volume of a pneumothorax approximates to the ratio of the cube of the lung diameter to the hemithorax diameter. This volume of pneumothorax can be calculated in percentage [36]. Some guidelines from the USA estimated the volume of a pneumothorax by measuring the distance from the lung apex to the cupola, and some British guidelines estimated the volume by measuring the interpleural distance at level of the hilum [29]. Pneumothorax size calculations are best achieved by CT scanning but are only recommended for difficult cases [36].

5. Treatment

Primary spontaneous pneumothorax can be treated conservatively or by intervention that include simple aspiration, chest tube drainage, thoracoscopy, and thoracotomy [37]. A lot of issues must be taken into consideration in the management of spontaneous pneumothorax. Studies have shown numerous approaches offered by different guidelines and associations. According to the American College of Chest Physicians (ACCP), the British Thoracic Society (BTS), and the Spanish Society of Pulmonology and Thoracic Surgery, the initial management of the primary spontaneous pneumothorax is directed to remove air from the pleural space and prevent recurrences [1, 38]. Treatment options for primary spontaneous pneumothorax go from simple observation, aspiration with a catheter, insertion of a chest tube, pleurodesis, thoracoscopy, video-assisted thoracoscopic surgery (which is one of the most studied approaches) to thoracotomy. Selection of the appropriate approach depends on the size of the pneumothorax, the severity of the symptoms, and the presence or absence or persistent air leak (**Figure 2**). An initial step in the management of primary spontaneous pneumothorax is to evaluate the patient hemodynamic stability and risk. When the patient is hemodynamically unstable and/or the pneumothorax is bilateral, chest drain should be performed. If the patient is hemodynamically stable, different approaches can be chosen [38].

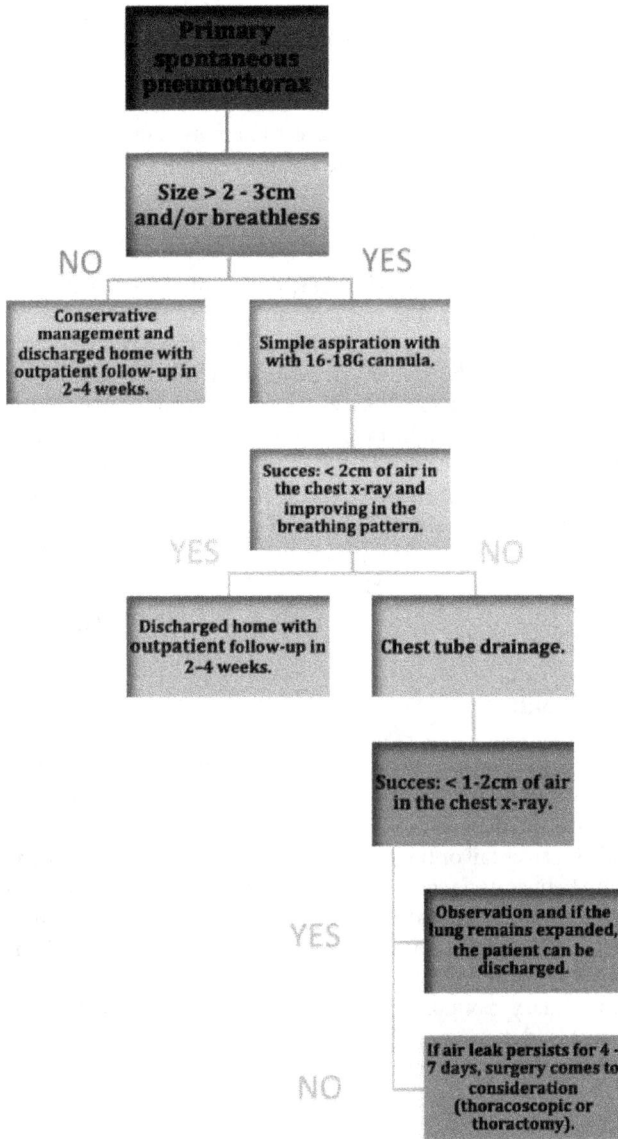

Figure 2.
Management of primary spontaneous pneumothorax [29].

5.1 Conservative management

Clinically stable patients with small pneumothoraces can be treated with conservative management, and they should stay in the emergency room with a control chest radiograph to perceive the resolution of pneumothorax. Conservative management consists of observing the patient, oxygen therapy, and analgesia [39]. In the case of symptomatic and/or large pneumothoraces, it is indicated to remove the air from the pleural space by simple aspiration or chest tube drainage [40]. Patients with a first episode of primary spontaneous pneumothorax that are hemodynamically stable, with few or no symptoms, and have a small pneumothorax (<2–3 centimeters between the lung and the chest wall or <15% of hemithorax) can be treated by supplemental oxygen, which accelerates the process of reabsorption of air by the pleura. The observation period should be at least 6 hours; after this time, the patient can be discharged if three conditions are met: absence of progression of the pneumothorax confirmed by a control chest radiograph, compliance of the outpatient treatment plans, and ease of access to emergency medical services. In these cases, the follow-up after discharge should be from 2 to 4 weeks [41].

5.2 Aspiration

Patients with a first episode of primary spontaneous pneumothorax episode, which are hemodynamically stable and have a large pneumothorax (more than 2–3 centimeters of air in chest X-ray or more than 15% of the hemithorax) or those who have a progressive pneumothorax, or symptomatic with chest pain, or dyspnea should undergo needle aspiration [29, 42]. Several methods are used to perform simple aspiration, ranging from intravenous catheters in the second intercostal space in the midclavicular line with 16–18G cannula to chest tubes that can be removed once re-expansion of the lung is confirmed [43]. When the procedure is successful (less than 2 centimeters of air in the chest X-ray and improving in the breathing pattern), the patient can be discharged, with follow-up from 2 to 4 weeks. Simple aspiration is successful in 70% of the patients with moderate-sized primary pneumothorax; in patients older than 50 years or aspirations bigger than 2.5 liters, this method is likely to fail [38].

5.3 Thoracostomy only

Primary spontaneous pneumothorax may also be managed with a chest tube that is left in place for 1 or more days or by attaching the catheter to a one-way Heimlich valve or water-seal device and using it as a chest tube. The last method is reserved for patients in whom Heimlich valves fail or those who have coexisting respiratory conditions that reduce the ability to tolerate a recurrent pneumothorax [38]. After treatment, persistent air leaks are not common in primary spontaneous pneumothorax. Seventy five percent of air leaks resolve after 7 days, and 100% resolve after 15 days [38]. When the air leak persists for 4 to 7 days, surgery comes to consideration. In a study from Kim, selection of patients with primary spontaneous pneumothorax and persistent air leaks for immediate surgery must be done according to the presence or absence of bullae, detected by high-resolution chest computed tomographic (HRCT) scanning [44].

5.4 Pleurodesis

The American College of Chest Physicians, British Thoracic Society, and the Belgian Society of Pulmonology recommended surgical pleurodesis via thoracoscopy for air leak that persists more than 4 days or recurrence prevention at second occurrence [45]. Methods of pleurodesis have included mechanical abrasion with gauze or Marlex, instillation of tetracycline, pleural irritation with laser or cautery, and instillation of talc [46]. The addition of pleurodesis agents reduces the rate of recurrence in PSP. Alayouty et al. in a randomized controlled trial studied the efficacy of different pleurodesis agents. They reported that chemical pleurodesis is associated with less recurrence rate than mechanical abrasion (P < 0.001, evidence level 1b) [47, 48].

5.5 Video-assisted thoracoscopic surgery (VATS)

The thoracoscopic surgery for primary spontaneous pneumothorax has been proposed and studied by a lot of clinicians as the main treatment for recurrent or persistent spontaneous pneumothorax. Surgical treatment is more invasive and has a lower recurrence rate than the conservative treatment [49–51] but increases patient discomfort, which has restricted the application of open thoracotomy. Video-assisted thoracoscopic surgery (VATS) for primary spontaneous pneumothorax has been proposed as a new surgical technique and has taken over the role of open thoracotomy, due to its minimal invasiveness and low morbidity [52]. This technique has been used not only for prolonged air leak or recurrence but also in patients at the first episode of pneumothorax, when blebs or bullae are identified with CT scan. A study conducted at the Chest Diseases Hospital in Kuwait treated spontaneous pneumothorax in 72 patients using VATS technique. The study included 67 male and 5 female patients from 15 to 40 years with a recurrent episode of pneumothorax. Surgeons performed VATS unilateral technique in all cases, with gauze abrasion and apical pleurectomy to remove subpleural blebs or bullae and excision of the apex of the upper lobe in the absence of any identifiable lesion. They concluded that thoracoscopic surgery could be carried out safely and effectively in the treatment of recurrent or persistent spontaneous pneumothorax, allowing inspection of the entire lung, identification of bullae, and resection of the bullous disease [29]. Another study compared the results of conservative treatment, open thoracotomy, and VATS. The authors studied 281 patients who had primary spontaneous pneumothorax, finding recurrences in 56.4% of the patients with the conservative treatment, 3% for open thoracotomy and 11.7% for VATS with a hospital stay length of 14.5, 22.2, and 8.3 days, respectively. At the end, they concluded VATS was significantly superior to open thoracotomy measuring length of operation, bleeding volume, and length of hospital stay. In terms of morbidity, low invasive and cosmetic issue VATS is superior to open thoracotomy [52]. Conventional three-port VATS has advantage in hospital stay, postoperative pain, and chest drainage time. In 2005, Dr. Gaetano Rocco used simple-port VATS for the first time, a technique that requires a minimum incision of approximately 3 cm and facilitates the postoperative recovery of the patient, compared with three-port VATS [53].

5.6 Open thoracotomy

Thoracotomy is an incision into the pleural space of the chest, and it has been the classic surgical treatment of PSP. Surgery is indicated when there is a recurrence of an initial episode of PSP, which produces persistent air leaks, or collapsed lung after placement of pleural drainage [54]. The advantages of this procedure over thoracoscopic techniques are the ability to perform extensive mechanical pleurodesis and the resection of blebs [55]. In order to prevent recurrence of pneumothorax, segments of the lung with bullae or blebs need to be resected. In 1941, Tyson and Grandall described open thoracotomy with pleural abrasion for the treatment of pneumothorax, and then Gaensler introduced parietal pleurectomy and less invasive procedures (like axillary thoracotomy); this became more common during the last years [56].

After the surgical treatment, the next step is to prevent the recurrence of spontaneous pneumothorax, which is estimated from 23 to 50% of all the patients. The highest risk occurs in the first 30 days, and, during this time, patients must avoid activities which involve acute variation of the pressure in the lungs, like flying or diving; these activities increase the risk of recurrent spontaneous pneumothorax. The recommendation for patients with the first episode of spontaneous pneumothorax is to avoid flying or diving. Patients may be able to fly 6 weeks after a definitive surgical intervention and resolution of the pneumothorax and after treatment; patients must perform a control X-ray to confirm the resolution and wait at least 6 weeks before flying. Recurrence of spontaneous pneumothorax is not common during a flight, but the consequences could be dangerous because there is not medical attention. Passengers may wish to consider alternative forms of transport within 1 year of the initial event [57]. The management of pneumothorax during a flight depends on the patient's clinical condition and the medical supplies on the plane. Supplemental oxygen should be provided, and the descent to the nearest airport considered [58].

6. Conclusion

PSP is a common problem encountered by doctors in medical practice. It is a significant global health problem affecting adolescent and young adults mainly. Current guidelines recommend treatment based on the severity of symptoms and the degree of lung collapse according to chest X-ray findings. There is an update needed in the current international guidelines including randomized controlled evidence. The first step in the management is to remove air from pleural space, with subsequent management aimed to prevent recurrence. Observation with supplemental oxygen, aspiration of intrapleural air, tube thoracostomy, and VATS pleurodesis with talc to prevent recurrence are the pillars of treatment. Thoracotomy should be reserved for special cases in which the patient is unable or unwilling to undergo VATS, in situations where VATS has failed or in high-risk cases.

Author details

Fabian Andres Giraldo Vallejo*, Rubby Romero, Melissa Mejia
and Estefania Quijano
Instituto del Corazon de Bucaramanga, Bucaramanga, Colombia

*Address all correspondence to: fabiangiraldomd@gmail.com

IntechOpen

References

[1] Wong A, Galiabovitch E, Bhagwat K. Management of primary spontaneous pneumothorax: A review: Management of spontaneous pneumothorax. ANZ Journal of Surgery [Internet]. 2018 Jul 5 [cited 2018 Sep 28]. Available from: http://doi.wiley.com/10.1111/ans.14713

[2] Henry M, Arnold T, Harvey J. BTS Guidelines for the Management of Spontaneous Pneumothorax. Thorax. 2003 May;**58**(Suppl 2):ii39-52

[3] Simpson G. Spontaneous pneumothorax: Time for some fresh air. Internal Medicine Journal. 2010 Mar;**40**(3):231-234

[4] Sahn SA. Spontaneous pneumothorax. The New England Journal of Medicine. 2000;7

[5] Bintcliffe O, Maskell N. Spontaneous pneumothorax. BMJ. 2014 May 8;**348**:g2928-g2928

[6] Brown SGA, Ball EL, Macdonald SPJ, Wright C, McD Taylor D. Spontaneous pneumothorax; A multicentre retrospective analysis of emergency treatment, complications and outcomes: Spontaneous pneumothorax. Internal Medicine Journal. 2014 May;**44**(5):450-457

[7] Tschopp J-M, Bintcliffe O, Astoul P, Canalis E, Driesen P, Janssen J, et al. ERS task force statement: Diagnosis and treatment of primary spontaneous pneumothorax. The European Respiratory Journal. 2015 Aug;**46**(2):321-335

[8] Massongo M, Leroy S, Scherpereel A, Vaniet F, Dhalluin X, Chahine B, et al. Outpatient management of primary spontaneous pneumothorax: A prospective study. The European Respiratory Journal. 2014 Feb 1;**43**(2):582-590

[9] Chen J-S, Chan W-K, Tsai K-T, Hsu H-H, Lin C-Y, Yuan A, et al. Simple aspiration and drainage and intrapleural minocycline pleurodesis versus simple aspiration and drainage for the initial treatment of primary spontaneous pneumothorax: An open-label, parallel-group, prospective, randomised, controlled trial. The Lancet. 2013 Apr;**381**(9874):1277-1282

[10] Noppen M, Alexander P, Driesen P, Slabbynck H, Verstraeten A. Manual aspiration versus chest tube drainage in first episodes of primary spontaneous pneumothorax: A multicenter, prospective, randomized pilot study. American Journal of Respiratory and Critical Care Medicine. 2002 May;**165**(9):1240-1244

[11] Sedrakyan A, van der MJ, Lewsey J, Treasure T. Video assisted thoracic surgery for treatment of pneumothorax and lung resections: Systematic review of randomised clinical trials. BMJ. 2004 Oct 30;**329**(7473):1008

[12] Margolis M, Gharagozloo F, Tempesta B, Trachiotis GD, Katz NM, Alexander EP. Video-assisted thoracic surgical treatment of initial spontaneous pneumothorax in young patients. The Annals of Thoracic Surgery. 2003 Nov;**76**(5):1661-1664

[13] Foroulis CN. Surgery for primary spontaneous pneumothorax. Journal of Thoracic Disease. 2016 Dec;**8**(12):E1743-E1745

[14] Chen Y-Y, Huang H-K, Chang H, Lee S-C, Huang T-W. Postoperative predictors of ipsilateral and contralateral recurrence in patients with primary spontaneous pneumothorax. Journal of Thoracic Disease. 2016 Nov;**8**(11):3217-3224

[15] Zarogoulidis K, Papaiwannou A, Lazaridis G, Karavergou A, Lampaki S, Baka S, et al. Pneumothorax from

Diagnosis to Treatment, Hands on Course: Part II. Annals of Translational Medicine. 2015 Mar;**3**(3):41. DOI: 10.3978/j.issn.2305-5839.2015.02.10

[16] Noppen M, De Keukeleire T. Pneumothorax. Respiration. 2008;**76**(2):121-127

[17] Bense L, Eklund G, Wiman L-G. Smoking and the increased risk of contracting spontaneous pneumothorax. Chest. 1987 Dec;**92**(6):1009-1012

[18] Iii LJM, Hepper NGG, Offord KP. Incidence of Spontaneous Pneumothorax in Olmsted County, Minnesota: 1950 to 1974. p. 4

[19] Sadikot RT, Greene T, Meadows K, Arnold AG. Recurrence of primary spontaneous pneumothorax. Thorax. 1997 Sep 1;**52**(9):805-809

[20] Guo Y, Xie C, Rodriguez RM, Light RW. Factors related to recurrence of spontaneous pneumothorax. Respirology. 2005 Jun;**10**(3):378-384

[21] Bobbio A, Dechartres A, Bouam S, Damotte D, Rabbat A, Régnard J-F, et al. Epidemiology of spontaneous pneumothorax: Gender-related differences. Respiratory Epidemiology. Thorax. 2015 Jul;**70**(7):653-658. DOI: 10.1136/thoraxjnl-2014-206577. Epub 2015 Apr 27

[22] Johnson MM. Catamenial pneumothorax and other thoracic manifestations of endometriosis. Clinics in Chest Medicine. 2004 Jun;**25**(2):311-319

[23] Hopkins TG, Maher ER, Reid E, Marciniak SJ. Recurrent pneumothorax. The Lancet. 2011 May;**377**(9777):1624

[24] Alifano M, Forti Parri SN, Bonfanti B, Arab WA, Passini A, Boaron M, et al. Atmospheric pressure influences the risk of pneumothorax. Chest. 2007 Jun;**131**(6):1877-1882

[25] Noppen M. Music: A new cause of primary spontaneous pneumothorax. Thorax. 2004 Aug 1;**59**(8):722-724

[26] Viveiro C, Rocha P, Carvalho C, Zarcos MM. Spontaneous pneumothorax as manifestation of Marfan syndrome. Case Reports. 2013 Dec 5;**2013**(Dec 05 1):bcr2013201697

[27] Karpman C, Aughenbaugh GL, Ryu JH. Pneumothorax and bullae in Marfan syndrome. Respiration. 2011;**82**(3):219-224

[28] Leite M de FMP, Aoun NBT, Borges MS, Magalhães MEC, Christiani LA. Marfan's syndrome: Early and severe form in siblings. Arquivos Brasileiros de Cardiologia. 2003 Jul;**81**(1):89-92

[29] MacDuff A, Arnold A, Harvey J, On behalf of the BTS Pleural Disease Guideline Group. Management of spontaneous pneumothorax: British Thoracic Society pleural disease guideline 2010. Thorax. 2010 Aug 1;**65**(Suppl 2):ii18-ii31

[30] Walker SP, Bibby AC, Halford P, Stadon L, White P, Maskell NA. Recurrence rates in primary spontaneous pneumothorax: A systematic review and meta-analysis. The European Respiratory Journal. 2018 Sep;**52**(3):1800864

[31] Roberts DJ, Leigh-Smith S, Faris PD, Blackmore C, Ball CG, Robertson HL, et al. Clinical presentation of patients with tension pneumothorax: A systematic review. Annals of Surgery. 2015 Jun;**261**(6):1068-1078

[32] Norris RM, Jones JG, Bishop JM. Respiratory gas exchange in patients with spontaneous pneumothorax. Thorax. 1968 Jul 1;**23**(4):427-433

[33] Glazer HS, Anderson DJ, Wilson BS, Molina PL, Sagel SS. Pneumothorax: Appearance on lateral chest radiographs. Radiology. 1989 Dec 1;**173**(3):707-711

[34] Terzi E, Zarogoulidis K, Kougioumtzi I, Dryllis G, Pitsiou G, Machairiotis N, et al. Acute respiratory distress syndrome and pneumothorax. Journal of Thoracic Disease. 2014;**6**:8

[35] Zhang M, Liu Z-H, Yang J-X, Gan J-X, Xu S-W, You X-D, et al. Rapid detection of pneumothorax by ultrasonography in patients with multiple trauma. **10**(4):7

[36] Hoi K, Turchin B, Kelly A-M. How accurate is the Light index for estimating pneumothorax size? Australasian Radiology. 2007 Apr;**51**(2):196-198

[37] Ashby M, Haug G, Mulcahy P, Ogden KJ, Jensen O, Walters JA. Conservative versus interventional management for primary spontaneous pneumothorax in adults. 2014;**17**

[38] Soulsby T. British Thoracic Society guidelines for the management of spontaneous pneumothorax: Do we comply with them and do they work? Emergency Medicine Journal. 1998 Sep 1;**15**(5):317-321

[39] Baumann MH, Noppen M. Pneumothorax. Respirology. 2004 Jun;**9**(2):157-164

[40] Leyn PD, Lismonde M, Ninane V, Noppen M, Slabbynck H, Meerhaeghe AV, et al. Belgian Society of Pneumology. Guidelines on the management of spontaneous pneumothorax. Acta Chirurgica Belgica. 2005 Jan;**105**(3):265-267

[41] Kelly A-M, Kerr D, Clooney M. Outcomes of emergency department patients treated for primary spontaneous pneumothorax. Chest. 2008 Nov;**134**(5):1033-1036

[42] Ho KK, Ong MEH, Koh MS, Wong E, Raghuram J. A randomized controlled trial comparing minichest tube and needle aspiration in outpatient management of primary spontaneous pneumothorax. The American Journal of Emergency Medicine. 2011 Nov;**29**(9):1152-1157

[43] Miller AC. Guidelines for the Management of Spontaneous Pneumothorax. p. 3

[44] Kim J, Kim K, Shim YM, Chang WI, Park K-H, Jun T-G, et al. Video-assisted thoracic surgery as a primary therapy for primary spontaneous pneumothorax: Decision making by the guideline of high-resolution computed tomography. Surgical Endoscopy. 1998 Nov;**12**(11):1290-1293

[45] Hallifax RJ, Yousuf A, Jones HE, Corcoran JP, Psallidas I, Rahman NM. Effectiveness of chemical pleurodesis in spontaneous pneumothorax recurrence prevention: A systematic review. Thorax. 2017 Dec;**72**(12):1121-1131

[46] Ayed AK, Al-Din HJ. The results of Thoracoscopic surgery for primary spontaneous pneumothorax. Chest. 2000 Jul;**118**(1):235-238

[47] Jouneau S, Sohier L, Desrues B. Pleurodesis for primary spontaneous pneumothorax. The Lancet. 2013 Jul;**382**(9888):203

[48] Alayouty HD, Hasan TM, Alhadad ZA, Omar Barabba R. Mechanical versus chemical pleurodesis for management of primary spontaneous pneumothorax evaluated with thoracic echography. Interactive CardioVascular and Thoracic Surgery. 2011 Nov 1;**13**(5):475-479

[49] Mouroux J, Elkaïm D, Padovani B, Myx A, Perrin C, Rotomondo C, et al. Video-assisted thoracoscopic treatment of spontaneous pneumothorax: Technique and results of one hundred cases. The Journal of Thoracic and Cardiovascular Surgery. 1996 Aug;**112**(2):385-391

[50] Liu H-P, Lin PJ, Hsieh M-J, Chang J-P, Chang C-H. Thoracoscopic

surgery as a routine procedure for spontaneous pneumothorax. Chest. 1995 Feb;**107**(2):559 562

[51] Sawada S, Watanabe Y, Moriyama S. Video-assisted thoracoscopic surgery for primary spontaneous pneumothorax. Chest. 2005 Jun;**127**(6):2226-2230

[52] Janssen J, Cardillo G. Primary spontaneous pneumothorax: Towards outpatient treatment and abandoning chest tube drainage. Respiration. 2011;**82**(2):201-203

[53] Xu W, Wang Y, Song J, Mo L, Jiang T. One-port video-assisted thoracic surgery versus three-port video-assisted thoracic surgery for primary spontaneous pneumothorax: A meta-analysis. Surgical Endoscopy. 2017 Jan;**31**(1):17-24

[54] Freixinet JL, Canalís E, Juliá G, Rodriguez P, Santana N, de Castro FR. Axillary thoracotomy versus videothoracoscopy for the treatment of primary spontaneous pneumothorax. The Annals of Thoracic Surgery. 2004 Aug;**78**(2):417-420

[55] Murray KD, Matheny RG, Howanitz EP, Myerowitz PD. A limited axillary thoracotomy as primary treatment for recurrent spontaneous pneumothorax. Chest. 1993 Jan;**103**(1):137-142

[56] Lazopoulos A, Barbetakis N, Lazaridis G, Baka S, Mpoukovinas I, Karavasilis V, et al. Open thoracotomy for pneumothorax. Journal of Thoracic Disease. 2015;7:6

[57] Managing passengers with respiratory disease planning air travel: British Thoracic Society recommendations. Thorax. 1 Apr 2002;**57**(4):289-304

[58] Hu X, Cowl CT, Baqir M, Ryu JH. Air travel and pneumothorax. Chest. 2014 Apr;**145**(4):688-694

Chapter 3

Video-Assisted Thoracoscopy in the Management of Primary and Secondary Pneumothorax

Kostantinos Poulikidis, Lee Gerson, John Costello and Wickii T. Vigneswaran

Abstract

The management of primary and secondary spontaneous pneumothorax can have many variations depending on the surgeons and their expertise of practice. The end goal is to stop the recurrence. The history of treatment, clinical indications for surgery, and preoperative and postoperative decision-making for intervention are summarized. Surgical intervention plays an important role in the management of recurrent pneumothorax and complex initial pneumothorax. Over the years the surgical techniques have evolved, and currently, video-assisted thoracoscopic techniques are frequently used in the management. In this concise report, we attempt to analyze the surgical techniques currently in use and their outcomes. Furthermore, we attempt to integrate future innovations in the management of this common disorder.

Keywords: pneumothorax, video-assisted thoracoscopy, pleurodesis, thoracotomy

1. Background

Pneumothorax is a diverse entity with a wide array of clinical etiologies. It is more common in men than women [1–4]. Although pneumothorax can be defined simply as an abnormal collection of air in the pleural space, in order to accurately classify pneumothorax, it is helpful to group it broadly as either spontaneous or traumatic in nature [1, 2]. Overall, traumatic causes of pneumothorax account for greater than 50% of pneumothoraces on an annual basis [3]. These include injuries due to either true penetration or blunt traumatic events, including gunshot wounds, stabbings, blunt force trauma to the chest, or iatrogenic traumas sustained as part of medical procedures, such as central venous catheter placement, needle biopsies, and thoracentesis. Outside of trauma, the remainders of pneumothoraces are classified as spontaneous in nature. Although spontaneous pneumothorax accounts for less than half of all pneumothoraces, this type of pneumothorax is often the one that most demands the ongoing attention of the thoracic surgeon in the acute setting.

Spontaneous pneumothorax is itself classified into primary and secondary etiologies. Primary spontaneous pneumothorax is any pneumothorax that occurs without any identifiable inciting event in a patient without any known lung disease. Secondary spontaneous pneumothorax, on the other hand, defines any pneumothorax that develops in a patient as a complication of known underlying lung disease. Many diseases of the lung parenchyma can cause clinical pneumothorax; those

IntechOpen

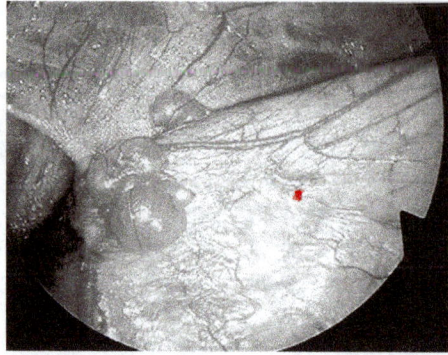

Figure 1.
Subpleural blebs of the apical lung with adhesion to the chest wall.

most commonly associated with its development include necrotizing pneumonias, cystic fibrosis, chronic obstructive pulmonary disease, and malignancy. Chronic obstructive pulmonary disease is the cause of 50–70% of all secondary spontaneous pneumothoraces. Catamenial pneumothorax is a very interesting clinical entity that is another, although rare, type of secondary spontaneous pneumothorax.

It is important to note that despite the definition of primary spontaneous pneumothorax indicating that it occurs in the setting of patients with no known lung disease, this is not completely clinically accurate. The majority of these patients do in fact have underlying lung disease with subpleural blebs (**Figure 1**), and it is the spontaneous rupture of these blebs that leads to the development of their pneumothoraces [3]. Despite a wide array of potential clinical etiologies, the overall incidence of spontaneous pneumothorax has been estimated at 17–24/100,000 in males and 1–6/100,000 in the female population [1–3]. Smoking increases the risk of contracting a first pneumothorax approximately 9-fold among women and 22-fold among men [5]. Spontaneous pneumothorax recurrence rates were similar for both men and women, with approximately 26% of patients experiencing a recurrence within 5 years of initial pneumothorax diagnosis [6].

2. History

The management of pneumothorax has seen large advancements over the past few decades. Surgical management of the disease did not begin until the 1940s when it was first documented by Tyson and Crandall in 1941 [7]. Treatment at that time involved a traditional transaxillary thoracotomy with resection of blebs. Later addition of pleurectomy or pleurodesis became routine in these patients. In the early 1990s, with the introduction of video-assisted thoracoscopy and mechanical stapling, minimally invasive chest surgery began to become popular for a variety of indications [8]. As a matter of fact, video-assisted thoracoscopic surgery (VATS) was first documented for pneumothorax [9]. Subsequently, VATS blebectomy, with the addition of pleurodesis or pleurectomy, began to take on popularity and remains often the choice of many. It was also demonstrated that VATS is superior to conservative treatment soon after [10].

3. Indications

Failure of conservative management and recurrence of pneumothorax are the most frequent indications for surgical intervention. In spontaneous pneumothorax, a large number of first episodes will be treated conservatively with non-operative intervention. Asymptomatic, small pneumothorax (less than 2 cm) can typically be observed with serial imaging. Larger symptomatic episodes need to be treated by drainage with needle decompression or with a chest tube. However, when the first episode is complicated and the pneumothoraces are unlikely to resolve using conservative management, surgical intervention may be necessary. These pneumothoraces include those complicated by hemothorax, bilaterality, persistent air leaks, or the inability of the lung to re-expand with conservative treatment [11–13].

4. Management

Recurrence rates for primary and secondary pneumothorax, when the initial episode was treated with chest tube drainage, have been reported as high as 18% in primary and 40% in secondary pneumothoraces [13]. Review of inpatient-treated pneumothorax demonstrated approximately 75% of recurrent pneumothoraces, which occurred in the first year following the initial pneumothorax. The probability of recurrence varied, depending on age group and the presence of underlying lung disease. For example, male patients aged 15–34 years, with underlying chronic lung disorders, had the highest probability of recurrent pneumothorax within 5 years of initial pneumothorax (39.2% recurrence rate) [6]. Some centers have reported being aggressive with first episode pneumothorax by treating these first episodes with VATS, significantly decreasing the recurrence rate in these patients [13]. In the past, open thoracotomy was the mainstay of surgical treatment for spontaneous pneumothorax, but with the institution of video-assisted thoracoscopic treatments, the number of surgeons performing open cases has decreased significantly. The objective of each operation is to prevent recurrence by resecting apical bullae or other causative blebs and perform a pleurodesis so future pneumothoraxes are unlikely [14]. With the heavy adoption of VATS, studies have attempted to identify differences in results and morbidity between the VATS and open thoracotomy techniques. VATS intervention was found to have recurrences in 3.8% compared to 1.8% in thoracotomy patients [15]. One meta-analysis, analyzing 4 randomized and 25 nonrandomized trials, assessed the recurrence rates of minimally invasive approach versus open [16]. It was stated that despite a fourfold increase recurrence rate for minimally invasive approach, this method was used three times more commonly than open in the United Kingdom [16]. Importantly however, the complication rates and pain can be significantly higher with thoracotomy than VATS, advocating a minimally invasive approach [15–17]. Some attribute the increased recurrence rate associated with VATS to the decreased amount of adhesions created with the smaller incisions than thoracotomy [17]. The decision as to the appropriate approach for these operations should involve a discussion with the patient for an informed decision, taking into consideration the balance between recurrence against decreased pain and recovery time.

The technical approach to VATS treatment of spontaneous pneumothorax involves patients undergoing general anesthesia with one-lung ventilation. The first incision is typically placed in the fifth or sixth interspace in the midaxillary line. Two additional incisions can typically be made in the fourth interspace in the anterior axillary line, as well as the fifth interspace in the auscultatory triangle [18]. There have been modifications to this strategy over the years, with variations in the number of incisions ranging to as low as one incision (**Figure 2**). Novel new methods are also being discussed such as a subxiphoid uniport incision [19]. This type of incision is currently being studied to assess for a decrease in the amount of intercostal nerve injury that is typically observed with intercostal incisions.

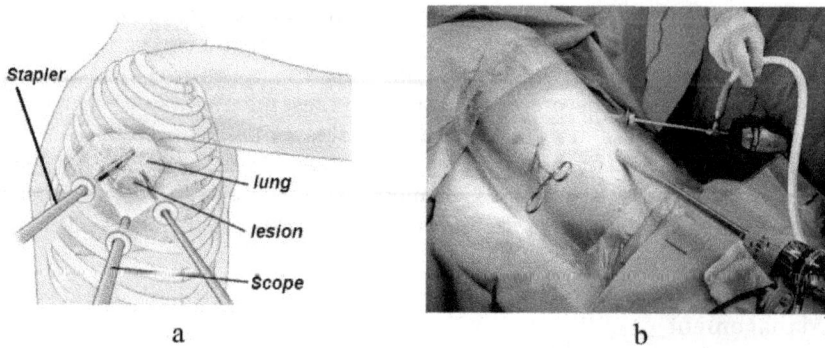

Figure 2.
Port placements for the classical three-port video-assisted thoracoscopic surgery. Different configurations, change according to the visual and staple requirements (a) camera through central port (b) Camera through posterior port.

Once safely in the chest, the lungs are carefully inspected to identify any bullous changes and to detect the source of the air leak. Blebs will be air-filled areas of the lung less than 1 cm in size compared to bullae which are greater than 1 cm in size. Adhesions should be identified and lysed to allow for complete evaluation of the lung. Care should be taken to obtain hemostasis if any bleeding from the adhesions is encountered. Bullae that are identified can be stapled using an endo-stapler without crossing over any portion of the bullae in the staple line, as this may increase risk of recurrence. There should be good margin with the stapler traversing only "healthy" lung tissue in patients with spontaneous primary pneumothorax.

Mechanical pleurodesis involves creating abrasions to the pleural surface, or performing a limited pleurectomy, to initiate an inflammatory response which results in the formation of adhesions and prevents the lung from collapsing in situations of recurrence. The pleural abrasion is typically performed using an electrocautery scratch pad or gauze (**Figure 3**). Care should be taken when working at the apex, as a Horner's syndrome can occur if there is any injury to the stellate ganglion of the sympathetic chain. Additional operative complications include bleeding, particularly from intercostal or mammary vessels, and pain. One randomized prospective study comparing wedge resection to wedge resection, and adjunct mechanical pleurodesis, resulted in no difference in recurrence rates but did show an increase in complications for the pleurodesis group [20]. A meta-analysis comparing the different combinations of intraoperative treatment for primary spontaneous pneumothorax found that wedge resection combined with chemical pleurodesis, as well as wedge resection, combined with both mechanical pleural abrasion and chemical pleurodesis, had the lowest recurrence rates. Although

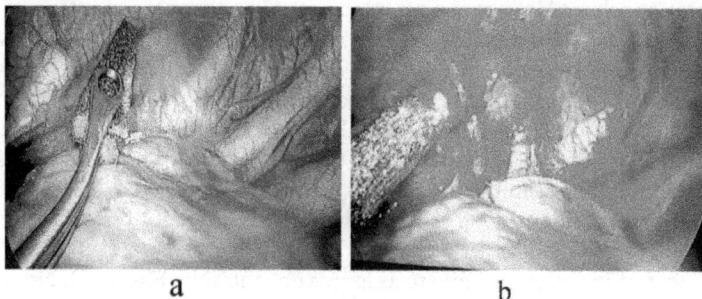

Figure 3.
Pleural abrasion using electrocautery scratch pad (a) before and (b) after.

the complications of these procedures were not taken into account favoring chemical or mechanical pleurodesis, in addition to wedge resection to remove the source of the air leak [21, 22]. Mechanical pleurodesis should be considered on a case-by-case basis with good clinical judgment. This should be avoided in patient who may have a bleeding tendency either due to medications or underlying disease. A chemical pleurodesis would be appropriate using an agent that cause aseptic inflammation in the pleura and facilitate pleural adhesion. Debate continues over the most effective chemical pleurodesis agent to use which has led to the widest variation in overall technique among all of these strategies. Graduated talcum of particle size <10 mic m is the most popular currently and has a long-standing history as an effective and trusted agent for pleurodesis. In the past, tetracycline and doxycycline have been used; however, the success rate is lower than the graduated talcum powder [23–25]. Marcheix et al. published a large study of 603 consecutive patients who underwent VATS pleurodesis using silver nitrate for primary spontaneous pneumothorax. While only 39.6% of these cases involved wedge resection and pleurodesis, the recurrence rate at 1 month was 0.5% in this group. The last 250 patients were included in a longer-term follow-up (2.9 ± 2.3 years) in which the recurrence rate was approximately 1.1%; however, only 73% of patients were actually contacted and this represents 31% of the total study population [26]. While it is difficult to draw concrete conclusions from this study, it is clear that silver nitrate can be an effective pleurodesis agent. Similar studies exist showing minocycline to be an effective agent as well [27].

When comparing VATS to other treatment modalities, such as aspiration, chest tube drainage, and pleurodesis, a recent meta-analysis of all available randomized control trials showed that VATS had the most favorable results with regard to recurrence and hospitalization days [21, 22]. The addition of pleurodesis to VATS bullectomy compared to VATS bullectomy alone further decreases recurrence rates, although this strategy comes with associated complications that include pain [21, 22]. Given the increased complications that arise from pleurodesis, some novel attempts at replacing the procedure, and at the same time achieving the same goal of promoting adhesions, have been developed. The use of an absorbable cellulose mesh and fibrin glue that are placed over blebectomy staple lines has been studied as an alternative to pleurodesis, with promising results [28]. This technique has been found to be non-inferior in terms of recurrence rates when compared to pleurodesis and is without the complications of bleeding, pain, and Horner's syndrome that are associated with mechanical pleurodesis. The cost of these biological materials should be taken into consideration when the approach is sought. The use of autologous blood as a pleurodesis agent needs mention. Although various chemical agents all pose some risks, namely, significant pain or rarely development of acute respiratory distress syndrome, pleurectomy carries with it significant pain and bleeding. Autologous blood has been utilized in some instances with good success [29]. The majority of the literature on this topic involves using blood to treat persistent air leaks in the postoperative period. While this data cannot be directly utilized to construct guidelines for spontaneous pneumothorax, based on the body of evidence that exists, its reported efficacy is so compelling that one wonders if it could be similarly effective in this operative setting.

Chang and colleagues compared pleurodesis combined with wedge resection utilizing "needlescopic" VATS technique with apical pleurectomy [30]. It is accurate to think of this technique as analogous to VATS, one 12 mm port for standard VATS instruments and the chest tube to that needlescopic technique which combines three 3 mm ports for "mini" endograspers and a "needlescope." In addition to demonstrating that pleurectomy was technically feasible, utilizing needlescopy with comparable pain indices, duration of chest tube drainage, and hospital stay, it also suggested a lower recurrence rate, 0%, when compared to the abrasion group, 8.6%. Studies comparing traditional VATS to needlescopic technique are lacking; however, in this author's experience, the former can be completed easily with only two 5 mm and a 10 mm port, a similar total incision length to needlescopy with one less incision overall, and can even be accomplished with a single 5 mm and a single 10 mm port. This fact calls into question the benefit of this modification to traditional VATS.

Two additional trials demonstrating the superiority of pleurodesis with pleurectomy over abrasion are worth mentioning. Huh and colleagues performed a similar study of 207 consecutive patients who underwent VATS wedge and either apical pleurectomy or pleural abrasion at a single Korean institution [31]. Although the recurrence rate in the pleurectomy group was higher in this study at 9.1% than the previous study, it was still lower than that of the abrasion group, 12.8%, which reached statistical significance. The second study is from the pediatric literature and showed that when combined with apical bleb resection pleurectomy led to a significantly lower rate of pneumothorax recurrence when compared to pleural abrasion, 8.8 vs. 40%, in the management of spontaneous primary pneumothorax in teenage patients ranging from 14 to 17 years old [32]. It should be noted that although these were retrospective studies, the follow-up period for the VATS wedge with pleurectomy group in the two Asian studies was significantly longer than that of the wedge with abrasion group, raising the possibility that the recurrence rate in the latter group may be underreported.

Secondary pneumothorax in the majority includes patients with chronic obstructive pulmonary disease and emphysema. The underlying may have homogenous or heterogeneous emphysema, and identifying the area of air leak can be difficult except in patients with large bullous disease. Other surgical strategies have been developed for the approach of pneumothorax in this patient population. When patients present with extensive emphysema of the underlying lung, the strategies of lung volume reduction surgery may be applicable. Lung volume reduction surgery (LVRS) is well studied by the National Emphysema Treatment Trial (NETT). LVRS in selected patients with emphysema as a treatment modality improved quality of life and length of survival compared to medical therapy alone [33]. A comparison of LVRS to medical therapy identified higher early mortality rates in the surgical group than medical treatment alone, 7.9 vs. 1.3%, though overall mortality saw no difference. The surgical group was further broken down into minimally invasive versus median sternotomy, identifying comparable mortality rates between the two arms. When comparing exercise capacity between the surgical and medical groups, there was a significant difference 24 months after treatment in favor of surgery, improving 15% of patients compared to 3% in the medical treatment arm. Application of NETT trial findings is useful and can provide clarity when approaching a patient presenting with secondary pneumothorax with severe emphysema. Work-up on these patients often show low FEV1 values with high residual volumes and lung capacity. In these patients applying the principle of lung volume reduction to include the suspected areas, this will help to treat the secondary pneumothorax as well as improving overall outcome. However this patient population should be approached with care and best treated in centers with expertise in LVRS. Often the staple lines will require reinforcement, and additional adjunctive procedures may be necessary such as pleural tent to manage air leak (**Figure 4a**) [34].

Patients presenting with secondary pneumothorax with underlying fibrotic parenchymal pathology present additional challenges [35]. These lungs have poor compliance, and air leak management will require a different approach that may need sealants rather than resection and use of pleural tent to manage the air leak and the space (**Figure 4b**). Use of tissue sealants instead of stapling, or in addition to stapling, may be necessary if the patient is deemed a candidate for surgical intervention. If not a surgical candidate, conservative approach with chemical pleurodesis would be appropriate.

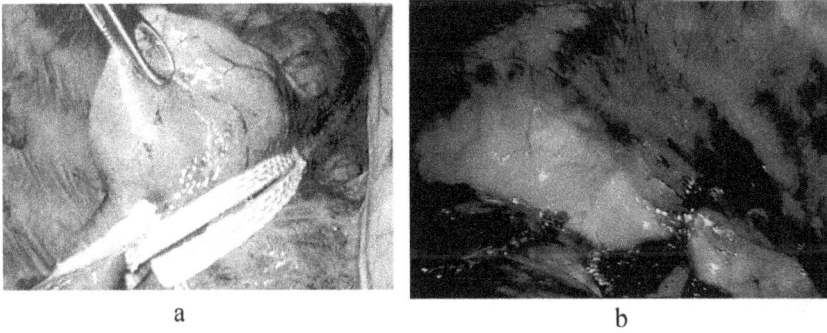

Figure 4.
(a) Using reinforcement techniques to reduce air leak at staple line and (b) using pleural tent to manage air leak and space in a noncompliant lung.

The most important consideration among patients with secondary spontaneous pneumothorax is that by definition, the patients are sicker than primary spontaneous pneumothorax patients because of the underlying lung condition at baseline. This lung pathology almost always accompanies in advanced age, with finding the mean age of patients presenting with primary spontaneous pneumothorax is younger than secondary pneumothorax. It stands to reason that this age brings with it more medical comorbidities and, as a result, reduced physiologic reserve, therefore necessitating prompt action, even when the size of the pneumothorax is relatively small. Furthermore, if one occurrence of pneumothorax in this patient population represents a life-threatening condition, then a recurrence could possibly be even more life-threatening. Therefore, one could argue that preventing recurrence of pneumothorax is more of a matter of life and death in secondary pneumothorax patient compared to primary spontaneous pneumothorax for the reasons listed above, as typically they have limited reserve [36, 37].

While agreement is coalescing that among patients treated with surgery for spontaneous pneumothorax, VATS should be the primary method of access. The diseased lung should be excised, and some form of pleurodesis should be added. Several other areas of interest warrant attention as well.

The strategy of postoperative chest tube management following surgical treatment for pneumothorax has not been extensively studied. Some surgeons advocate the placing of chest tubes to allow wall suction to increase the lung-chest wall apposition after pleurodesis, while others prefer to leave chest tubes on water seal in the immediate postoperative period. One study has compared these two strategies for chest tube management, demonstrating that placing patients on -20 cm H_2O suction resulted in increased chest tube duration, hospital stay, and prolonged air leak compared to those patients on no suction [38]. As long as pleural apposition is noted on chest radiograph postoperatively, the use of suction can be avoided that suggest prolonged air leak and subsequent hospital stay.

Some suggest that the cost and length of hospital stay might be reduced by instituting "clever" drainage strategies. One such approach is the use of digital electronic drainage systems to manage chest tubes. Removal of chest drains remains an important factor in timing of discharge from the hospital following lung resection. Since data was first published on the first digital suction device in 2006, there has been increased interest in the idea of utilizing objective data from these devices to dictate timing of the removal of chest drains, thereby reducing inter-operator variability and hopefully length of stay [39]. A group in Korea expanded on this idea by utilizing Wi-Fi-enabled digital suction devices in the postoperative management of chest drainage tubes in patients undergoing VATS wedge resection for primary spontaneous pneumothorax

[40]. The devices utilized in this study could not only remotely deliver information to providers regarding suction power and volume of air leaks, but they could also allow the providers to remotely control settings on the suction device. In keeping with the growing reliance on mobile technology in our society, clinicians were able to monitor and control device parameters using a smartphone app. Findings in this randomized control trial were consistent with previous studies which showed a statistically significant decrease in chest tube duration, length of stay, and, consequently, overall cost. The investigators established the safety and feasibility of managing pleural drains remotely opening the possibility of discharging patients home with the drains in place and monitoring their progress at home. One limitation of this particular study was that investigators elected not perform any form of pleurodesis to limit the postoperative parameters, thereby reducing the generalizability of the data onto patients who received the gold standard of treatment for spontaneous pneumothoraces, namely, resection and pleurodesis. Despite this limitation, recurrences in this study with 6 months of follow-up data remained low at about 3.4%. Given the rapidity with which mobile technology is advancing, it is not hard to envision a time when physicians can monitor the character and volume of effluent from these devices as well, thereby decreasing the need for inpatient care to that of reaching a stable level of analgesia with only oral agents.

There are also financial implications that should be considered when evaluating the differences between open and minimally invasive approaches to the management of pneumothorax and use of adjuncts. In a small Italian study from 1996 comparing VATS versus thoracotomy for management of recurrent spontaneous pneumothorax at a time when reusable VATS instruments were not yet widely available, VATS was still found to have a 22.7% cost savings compared to thoracotomy even when expensive disposable VATS equipment was used. The cost savings at that time were realized in the decreased duration of postoperative hospitalization seen in patients treated with VATS compared to open thoracotomy [10, 41]. A more recent study identified these cost savings in complication, ICU admission, length of hospitalization, operative time, and chest tube duration [42], further supporting the argument of minimally invasive intervention compared to open.

As application of robotic techniques become readily available to thoracic surgeons, it is likely the technology could be developed in pinpointing air leak and precision application of treatment during surgical intervention. Furthermore, there is an increasing interest in using computerized chest drainage systems to allow for an early and safe removal of chest tube or remote management of the tube in outpatient settings.

Anesthetic concerns are typically left out of discussion of surgical treatment. However, one paper that deserves mention evaluated the feasibility of performing awake VATS bullectomy and abrasion. In this randomized control trial in Rome, Italy, patients were randomized to undergo either awake VATS with thoracic epidural anesthesia or traditional VATS with general anesthesia and single-lung ventilation [43]. The sample size was relatively small to be sure, with 21 in the investigational arm and 23 in the control arm, but the results of the trial were striking nonetheless. Not only was awake VATS technically feasible, with all cases being completed as planned and zero conversions to general anesthesia, but pain scores and patient satisfaction with anesthesia favored the awake approach over the traditional VATS. What is particularly interesting in this study is that the cost data also favored the awake technique (2540 ± 352 € vs. 3550 ± 435 €, $p < 0.0001$). This is mostly because anesthesia time (25.0 ± 6.0 min vs. 35.5 ± 10.0 min, $p < 0.001$), recovery room time (20 ± 15.0 min vs. 30 ± 15.0 min, $p = 0.001$), global OR time (78.0 ± 20.0 min vs. 105.0 ± 15.0 min, $p < 0.001$), and hospital stay (2.0 ± 1.0 d vs. 3.0 ± 1.0 d, $p < 0.0001$) were all shorter for the awake group [43]. With a significant portion of the debate over how best to control rising health-care costs with focus on resource utilization and hospital stay, it is a wonder why this technique is not more widely utilized, let alone discussed.

The rise of minimally invasive surgical treatment of spontaneous pneumothorax has had a great impact on the way in which these are approached. Prior to the adoption of VATS techniques, many patients were deemed too sick to tolerate either single-lung ventilation or the ventilator assistance required in the perioperative period or both. Ichinose and colleagues retrospectively evaluated the records of all patients operated on for secondary pneumothorax, 183 cases, at a single institution between 1993 and 2014 and reported on the outcome of their surgical treatment [37]. Other than the underlying lung pathology, of which interstitial pneumonia had the worst survival, the group identified open surgical treatment as the greatest risk factor for treatment failure defined as the occurrence of in-hospital mortality, postoperative complications, and death within 6 months or ipsilateral recurrence within 2 years. In noting the dearth of evidence regarding minimally invasive surgical techniques for secondary pneumothorax, Galvez and colleagues highlight the promise of non-intubated VATS (NI-VATS) surgery in this population [44]. In addition to the benefits of this technique described above for PSP, the benefits of avoiding general anesthesia in these patients also include decreasing risk of ventilator dependency, decreasing risk of pulmonary infections, secretions of orotracheal intubation, and a reduction in overall pulmonary complications by half. Much of the pleurodesis reported in this literature review involved fibrin glue, polyglycolic acid sheets, and autologous blood or some combination of these. It seems obvious that because of the decreased physiologic and cardiopulmonary reserve often seen in patients with secondary pneumothorax, there should be great interest in developing additional minimally invasive surgical techniques and investigating their benefits.

5. Conclusion

Despite differences in etiology of pneumothorax, the management should be directed at expeditious bedside and, ultimately, surgical management for patients who do not completely resolve their pneumothorax non-operatively [45]. We advocate for bedside chest tube placement under local anesthetic for nearly all patients who present with spontaneous pneumothorax, except those with small pneumothorax that remain stable on follow-up radiographic imaging. Following chest tube placement, if the pneumothorax fully resolves and there is no ongoing air leak, these patients can have their chest tube water sealed and subsequently removed as early as the day after hospital presentation. Patients with recurrent bilateral pneumothorax, patients who present for the first time without ready access to medical care, patients with profession or hobbies that make them at higher risk from developing recurrence, or patients with persistent air leak should undergo surgical intervention whenever possible. The operative approach should favor VATS over open thoracotomy for both pleurodesis/pleurectomy and resection of blebs. Our approach is always to perform pleurodesis following the blebectomy or remove the source of the air leak. Our preferred approach in younger patients is mechanical pleurodesis, and in patients above 65 years of age, use graded talc. In patients presenting with recurrences following a previous pleurodesis, we reserve the apical pleurectomy. In patients with secondary pneumothorax, we have lower threshold to reinforce staple line or perform pleural tent in addition to the above. This overall strategy will facilitate timely treatment in this patient population and accomplish it in a minimally invasive manner that aligns with other modern surgical approaches in the field of thoracic surgery.

Conflict of interest

None.

Author details

Kostantinos Poulikidis*, Lee Gerson, John Costello and Wickii T. Vigneswaran
Loyola University Health System, Maywood, IL, USA

*Address all correspondence to: wickii.vigneswaran@lumc.edu

IntechOpen

References

[1] Onuki T, Ueda S, Yamaoka M, et al. Primary and secondary spontaneous pneumothorax: Prevalence, clinical features, and in-hospital mortality. Canadian Respiratory Journal. 2017;**2017**:1-8. DOI: 10.1155/2017/6014967

[2] Gupta D, Hansell A, Nichols T, Duong T, Ayres JG, Strachan D. Epidemiology of pneumothorax in England. Thorax. 2000;**55**(8):666-671. Available from: http://www.ncbi.nlm.nih.gov/pubmed/10899243

[3] Sahn SA, Heffner JE. Spontaneous pneumothorax. The New England Journal of Medicine. 2000;**342**(12):868-874. DOI: 10.1056/NEJM200003233421207

[4] Bobbio A, Dechartres A, Bouam S, et al. Epidemiology of spontaneous pneumothorax: Gender-related differences. Thorax. 2015;**70**(7):653-658

[5] Bense L, Eklund G, Wiman LG. Smoking and the increased risk of contracting spontaneous pneumothorax. Chest. 1987;**92**(6):1009-1012. DOI: 10.1378/chest.92.6.1009

[6] Hallifax RJ, Goldacre R, Landray MJ, et al. Trends in the incidence and recurrence of inpatient-treated spontaneous pneumothorax, 1968-2016. Journal of the American Medical Association. 2018;**320**(14):1471-1480. DOI: 10.1001/jama.2018.14299

[7] Tyson M, Crandall W. The surgical treatment of recurrent idiopathic spontaneous pneumothorax. The Journal of Thoracic Surgery. 1941;**10**:566-570

[8] Lewis RJ, Caccavale RJ, Sisler GE, Mackenzie JW. One hundred consecutive patients undergoing video-assisted thoracic operations. The Annals of Thoracic Surgery. 1992;**54**(3):421-426. Available from: http://www.ncbi.nlm.nih.gov/pubmed/1510508

[9] Levi JF, Kleinmann P, Riquet M, Debesse B. Percutaneous parietal pleurectomy for recurrent spontaneous pneumothorax. Lancet (London, England). 1990;**336**(8730):1577-1578. Available from: http://www.ncbi.nlm.nih.gov/pubmed/1979386

[10] Schramel FM, Sutedja TG, Braber JC, van Mourik JC, Postmus PE. Cost-effectiveness of video-assisted thoracoscopic surgery versus conservative treatment for first time or recurrent spontaneous pneumothorax. The European Respiratory Journal. 1996;**9**(9):1821-1825

[11] Lara-Guerra H, Waddell TK. Pearson's Thoracic and Esophageal Surgery. Philadelphia: Chirchill Livingstone; 2008. DOI: 10.1016/B978-0-443-06861-4.50014-9

[12] Schoenenberger RA, Haefeli WE, Weiss P, Ritz RF. Timing of invasive procedures in therapy for primary and secondary spontaneous pneumothorax. Archives of Surgery. 1991;**126**(6):764-766. Available from: http://www.ncbi.nlm.nih.gov/pubmed/2039365

[13] Hatz RA, Kaps MF, Meimarakis G, Loehe F, Müller C, Fürst H. Long-term results after video-assisted thoracoscopic surgery for first-time and recurrent spontaneous pneumothorax. The Annals of Thoracic Surgery. 2000;**70**(1):253-257. Available from: http://www.ncbi.nlm.nih.gov/pubmed/10921718

[14] Treasure T. Minimally invasive surgery for pneumothorax: The evidence, changing practice and current opinion. Journal of the Royal Society of Medicine. Sep 2007;**100**(9):419-422. DOI: 10.1258/jrsm.100.9.419

[15] Pagès PB, Delpy JP, Falcoz PE, et al. Videothoracoscopy versus thoracotomy for the treatment of spontaneous pneumothorax: A propensity score analysis. The Annals of Thoracic Surgery. 2015;**99**(1):258-263. DOI: 10.1016/j.athoracsur.2014.08.035

[16] Barker A, Maratos EC, Edmonds L, Lim E. Recurrence rates of video-assisted thoracoscopic versus open surgery in the prevention of recurrent pneumothoraces: A systematic review of randomised and non-randomised trials. Lancet. 28 Jul 2007;**370**(9584):329-335. DOI: 10.1016/S0140-6736(07)61163-5

[17] Sawada S, Watanabe Y, Moriyama S. Video-assisted thoracoscopic surgery for primary spontaneous pneumothorax: Evaluation of indications and long-term outcome compared with conservative treatment and open thoracotomy. Chest. 2005;**127**(6):2226-2230. DOI: 10.1378/chest.127.6.2226

[18] Cardillo G, Facciolo F, Giunti R, et al. Videothoracoscopic treatment of primary spontaneous pneumothorax: A 6-year experience. The Annals of Thoracic Surgery. 2000;**69**(2):357-361; discussion 361-2. Available from: http://www.ncbi.nlm.nih.gov/pubmed/10735663

[19] Li L, Tian H, Yue W, Li S, Gao C, Si L. Subxiphoid vs intercostal single-incision video-assisted thoracoscopic surgery for spontaneous pneumothorax: A randomised controlled trial. International Journal of Surgery. 2016;**30**:99-103. DOI: 10.1016/j.ijsu.2016.04.035

[20] Min X, Huang Y, Yang Y, et al. Mechanical pleurodesis does not reduce recurrence of spontaneous pneumothorax: A randomized trial. The Annals of Thoracic Surgery. Nov 2014;**98**(5):1790-1706. DOI: 10.1016/j.athoracsur.2014.06.034

[21] Sudduth CL, Shinnick JK, Geng Z, McCracken CE, Clifton MS, Raval MV. Optimal surgical technique in spontaneous pneumothorax: A systematic review and meta analysis. The Journal of Surgical Research. 2017. DOI: 10.1016/j.jss.2016.10.024

[22] Vuong NL, Elshafay A, Thao LP, et al. Efficacy of treatments in primary spontaneous pneumothorax: A systematic review and network meta-analysis of randomized clinical trials. Respiratory Medicine. 2018;**137**:152-166. DOI: 10.1016/j.rmed.2018.03.009

[23] Olsen PS, Anderson HO. Long term results after tetracycline pleurodesis in spontaneous pneumothorax. The Annals of Thoracic Surgery. 1992;**53**:1015-1017

[24] Kennedy L, Sahn SA. Talc pleurodesis for the treatment of pneumothorax and pleural effusion. Chest. 1994;**106**:1215-1222

[25] Maskell NA, Lee YC, Gleeson FV, Hedley EL, Pengelly G, Davies RJ. Randomized trials describing lung inflammation after pleurodesis with talc of varying particle size. American Journal of Respiratory and Critical Care Medicine. 2004;**170**(4):377-382. Epub 2004 May 13

[26] Marcheix B, Brouchet L, Renaud C, et al. Videothoracoscopic silver nitrate pleurodesis for primary spontaneous pneumothorax: An alternative to pleurectomy and pleural abrasion? The European Journal of Cardio-Thoracic Surgery. Jun 2007;**31**(6):1106-1109. DOI: 10.1016/j.ejcts.2007.03.017

[27] Chen JS, Chan WK, Tsai KT, et al. Simple aspiration and drainage and intrapleural minocycline pleurodesis versus simple aspiration and drainage for the initial treatment of primary spontaneous pneumothorax: An open-label, parallel-group, prospective, randomised, controlled trial. Lancet. 13 Apr 2013;**381**(9874):1277-1282. DOI: 10.1016/S0140-6736(12)62170-9

[28] Lee S, Kim HR, Cho S, et al. Staple line coverage after bullectomy for primary spontaneous pneumothorax: A randomized trial. The Annals of Thoracic Surgery. 2014;**98**(6):2005-2011. DOI: 10.1016/j.athoracsur.2014.06.047

[29] Pathak V, Quinn C, Zhou C, Wadie G. Use of autologous blood patch for prolonged air leak in spontaneous pneumothoraces in the adolescent population. Lung India. 2018;**35**(4): 328-331. DOI: 10.4103/lungindia.lungindia_462_17

[30] Chang YC, Chen CW, Huang SH, Chen JS. Modified needlescopic video-assisted thoracic surgery for primary spontaneous pneumothorax: The long-term effects of apical pleurectomy versus pleural abrasion. Surgical Endoscopy and Other Interventional Techniques. 2006;**20**(5):757-762. DOI: 10.1007/s00464-005-0275-6

[31] Huh U, Kim Y-D, Cho JS, Hoseok I, Lee JG, Lee JH. The effect of thoracoscopic pleurodesis in primary spontaneous pneumothorax: Apical parietal pleurectomy versus pleural abrasion. Korean Journal of Thoracic and Cardiovascular Surgery. 2012;**45**(5):316-319. DOI: 10.5090/kjtcs.2012.45.5.316

[32] Joharifard S, Coakley BA, Butterworth SA. Pleurectomy versus pleural abrasion for primary spontaneous pneumothorax in children. Journal of Pediatric Surgery. 2017. DOI: 10.1016/j.jpedsurg.2017.01.012

[33] Fishman A, Martinez F, Naunheim K, et al. A randomized trial comparing lung-volume-reduction surgery with medical therapy for severe emphysema. The New England Journal of Medicine. 2003;**348**(21):2059-2073. DOI: 10.1056/NEJMoa030287

[34] Vigneswaran WT, Podbielski FJ, Halldorsson A, Kong L, Schwab T, Janulitis C, et al. Single-stage, bilateral, video-assisted thoracoscopic lung volume reduction surgery for end-stage emphysema. World Journal of Surgery. 1998;**22**:799-802

[35] Nishimoto K, Fujisawa T, Yoshimura K, Enomoto Y, Enomoto N, Nakamura Y, et al. The prognostic significance of pneumothorax in patients with idiopathic pulmonary fibrosis. Respirology. 2017;**23**:519-525

[36] Isaka M, Asai K, Urabe N. Surgery for secondary spontaneous pneumothorax: Risk factors for recurrence and morbidity. Interactive Cardiovascular and Thoracic Surgery. 2013;**17**(2):247-252

[37] Ichinose J, Nagayama K, Hino H, Nitadori J, et al. Results of surgical treatment for secondary spontaneous pneumothorax according to underlying diseases. European Journal of Cardiothoracic Surgery. 2016;**49**(4):1132-1136. DOI: 10.1093/ejcts/ezv256

[38] Ayed AK. Suction versus water seal after thoracoscopy for primary spontaneous pneumothorax: Prospective randomized study. The Annals of Thoracic Surgery. 2003;**75**(5):1593-1596. Available from: http://www.ncbi.nlm.nih.gov/pubmed/12735584

[39] Pompili C, Detterbeck F, Papagiannopoulos K, et al. Multicenter international randomized comparison of objective and subjective outcomes between electronic and traditional chest drainage systems. The Annals of Thoracic Surgery. 2014;**98**(2):490-497. DOI: 10.1016/j.athoracsur.2014.03.043

[40] Cho HM, Hong YJ, Byun CS, Hwang JJ. The usefulness of Wi-Fi based digital chest drainage system in the post-operative care of pneumothorax. Journal of Thoracic Disease. 2016;**8**(3):396-402. DOI: 10.21037/jtd.2016.02.54

[41] Crisci R, Coloni GF. Video-assisted thoracoscopic surgery versus thoracotomy for recurrent spontaneous pneumothorax. A comparison of results and costs. European Journal of Cardio-Thoracic Surgery. 1996;**10**(7):556-560. Available from: http://www.ncbi.nlm.nih.gov/pubmed/8855429

[42] Joshi V, Kirmani B, Zacharias J. Thoracotomy versus VATS: Is there an optimal approach to treating pneumothorax? Annals of the Royal College of Surgeons of England. 2013;**95**(1):61-4.27

[43] Pompeo E, Tacconi F, Mineo D, Mineo TC. The role of awake video-assisted thoracoscopic surgery in spontaneous pneumothorax. The Journal of Thoracic and Cardiovascular Surgery. 2007;**133**(3):786-790. DOI: 10.1016/j.jtcvs.2006.11.001

[44] Galvez C, Bolufer S, Navarro-Martinez J, Lirio F, Corcoles JM, Rodriguez-Paniagua JM. Non-intubated video-assisted thoracic surgery management of secondary spontaneous pneumothorax. The Annals of Translational Medicine. 2015;**3**(8):104. DOI: 10.3978/j.issn.2305-5839.2015.04.24

[45] Vigneswaran WT, Odell JA. Pneumothorax: In Decision Making in Thoracic Surgery. New Delhi, India: Jaypee Brothers Medical Publishers Ltd; 2018. pp. 19-21

Chapter 4

Catamenial Pneumothorax

Sezai Celik and Ezel Erşen

Abstract

Catamenial pneumothorax is a rare condition in which spontaneous pneumothorax is recurrent. The incidence of catamenial pneumothorax has been
underestimated for a few number of reasons. Recently, the etiology of catamenial
pneumothorax has been more accurately diagnosed because of increased awareness and interest in the disease. Common and effective use of VATS technique
contributed to better understanding of the disease. The management of the disease
is difficult because of high recurrence rate. Operative and nonoperative interventions should be practiced more to prevent recurrences. Hormonal therapy should
be added to treatment in selected cases. In this chapter, we will discuss all aspects of
catamenial pneumothorax from diagnosis to treatment.

Keywords: pneumothorax, menstruation, catamenial, surgery

1. Introduction

Recurrent pneumothorax which is associated with menstruation is named as
"catamenial pneumothorax" (CPX). It was first reported by Maurer et al. [1] and
was presented to be a form of ectopic endometriosis and the term CPX was stated
by Lillington et al. [2].

"Catamenial" is a name from Greek meaning "monthly." CPX is most commonly
associated with endometriosis, but other etiological mechanisms of this disease
exist [3–6].

In the literature, CPX is defined to be a recurrent pneumothorax occurring up to
24 h before or within 72 h after the onset of menstruation [4, 6], and on the other
hand, not necessarily appearing every month [7]. Symptoms and signs of CPX are
mostly unspecific so much clinical suspicion has to be maintained [8]. CPX is a rare
entity; however, regarding literature, about one-third of all surgically treated cases
of pneumothorax in women are diagnosed to be CPX [9–12].

Therefore, thoracic endometriosis should always be suspected in reproductive-
age woman who suffer chest pain from spontaneous pneumothorax.

Thoracic endometriosis syndrome may be associated with other causes than pelvic endometriosis. In the first 24–48 h of menstruation, symptoms begin to appear
and are usually seen on the right side of the chest. In 90% of the patients, chest pain
is the most common symptom, and in one-third of the patients, shortness of breath
is rarely seen, but hemoptysis is also added to the clinical picture [13]. In the light of
these findings, the diagnosis of the disease is made clinically.

From 3 to 6% of spontaneous pneumothorax cases are catamenial pneumothorax, about one-third of all surgically treated cases of pneumothorax in affected
women.

The mean age of onset is reported to be 32–35 years [3, 4, 12, 14–17]. CPX may also develop as late as at 39 years of age [18, 19]. CPX occurs most often (85–95%) unilaterally, usually occurring on the right side of the chest, but there are cases on which pneumothorax also occurs on the left side or bilaterally [11, 15–21].

2. Incidence

CPX is generally considered to be a rare entity, and there is an incidence less than 3–6% among women who suffer from spontaneous pneumothorax. Such a low incidence rate may be a result of decreased disease awareness and underdiagnosis [4, 8–10, 19, 22–29].

Yet, the incidence of catamenial pneumothorax was much higher among women at reproductive age who were referred for surgical treatment because of recurrent spontaneous pneumothorax, ranging between 18 and 33% [9–12, 22].

In a recent study [24, 29, 30], 156 premenopausal women who underwent surgery for spontaneous pneumothorax were reviewed retrospectively, and 31.4% (49/156) of the patients were classified as CPX.

In a retrospective study, Alifano et al. reported thoracic endometriosis in 13 out of 35 (37%) patients who underwent reoperation for recurrent spontaneous pneumothorax [29]. Catamenial pneumothorax was the initial diagnosis in eight cases and idiopathic pneumothorax in four cases [29]. Under/misdiagnosis of thoracic endometriosis can be referred to several causes, including decreased disease awareness, incomplete scanning for the lesions, variations in the size, appearance, and number of the lesions [24, 30].

3. Etiology

The etiopathology of catamenial pneumothorax remains unclear, but there are some theories explaining the etiopathogenesis of catamenial pneumothorax. These theories include physiological, migrational, microembolic-metastatic, and the diaphragmatic theory of air passage [17] (**Table 1**).

According to the physiologic hypothesis, high levels of circulating prostaglandin F2 during menstrual cycle cause vasoconstriction and this induces alveolar rupture and pneumothorax. Pulmonary bullae blebs may be more sensitive to ruptures during hormonal changes. There are no pathognomonic lesions in such cases and this issue supports the physiologic theory [4, 7, 8, 24, 31].

In metastatic or lymphovascular microembolization theory, endometrial tissue spread through the venous and/or the lymphatic system to the lungs, and subsequent catamenial necrosis of endometrial parenchymal site adjacent to visceral pleura causes pneumothorax. If parenchymal endometrial focus is located centrally, hemoptysis may be present as a symptom [3, 4, 7, 8, 22, 24, 30–32]. Endometrial tissue can be detected in the lung parenchyma, at knee, in the brain, and in the eye. This supports the metastatic theory [12].

According to the transgenital-transdiaphragmatic passage of air theory, absence of cervical mucus during menstruation provides air passage from the vagina to the uterus, through the cervix. Then, air enters the peritoneal cavity straight through the fallopian tubes and reaches to the pleural space by diaphragmatic defects [4, 7, 8, 22, 24, 31]. This passage is facilitated by the difference in atmospheric pressures between pleural space and peritoneal space since the atmospheric pressure in the pleural cavity is less than the pressure in the peritoneal cavity.

Physiological hypothesis	High levels of circulating prostaglandin F2 during menstrual cycle cause vasoconstriction, and this induces alveolar rupture and pneumothorax.
Metastatic or lymphovascular microembolization hypothesis	Endometrial tissue spreads through the venous and/or the lymphatic system to the lungs, and subsequent catamenial necrosis of endometrial parenchymal site adjacent to visceral pleura causes pneumothorax
Transgenital-transdiaphragmatic passage of air hypothesis	Absence of cervical mucus during menstruation provides air passage from the vagina to the uterus, through the cervix. Then air enters the peritoneal cavity straight through the fallopian tubes and reaches to the pleural space by diaphragmatic defects.
Migration hypothesis	Following catamenial necrosis of this diaphragmatic endometrial implants results in diaphragmatic perforations. Endometrial tissue then passes through this diaphragmatic perforation and spreads into the thoracic cavity. Ectopic endometrial tissue implants to the visceral pleura and following catamenial necrosis of this tissue causes rupture of the underlying alveoli, and pneumothorax occurs.

These theories include physiological, migrational, microembolic-metastatic, and the diaphragmatic theory of air passage.

Table 1.
The etiopathology of catamenial pneumothorax remains unclear, but there are some theories explaining the etiopathogenesis of catamenial pneumothorax.

There are few reports in the literature regarding transgenital-transdiaphragmatic passage of air theory. There are rare cases reporting simultaneous [33, 34] or undulating episodes CPX and pneumoperitoneum [35], and also case reports defining radiologic findings of small diaphragmatic defects associated with ipsilateral CPX [21]. But repeated episodes of pneumothorax after hysterectomy, fallopian tube ligation, and diaphragmatic resection provide evidence that all the CPX cases can be explained by this theory [7, 24, 29, 36].

Migration theory is based on retrograde menstruation which causes in pelvic seeding of endometrial tissue and migration of this tissue to the subdiaphragmatic sites through the peritoneal fluid flow. Endometrial tissue is mostly implanted to the right hemidiaphragm because peritoneal circulation prefers a clockwise flow through the right paracolic gutter to right hemidiaphragm and the liver facilitates flow with its piston-like activity. Catamenial necrosis of this diaphragmatic endometrial implants results in diaphragmatic perforations. Endometrial tissue then passes through this diaphragmatic perforation and spreads into the thoracic cavity. Ectopic endometrial tissue implants to the visceral pleura and following catamenial necrosis of this tissue cause rupture of the underlying alveoli, and pneumothorax occurs [3, 4, 7, 8, 22, 24, 30, 31]. Endometrial diaphragmatic implants exist along with diaphragmatic perforations [37], and endometrial tissue can be seen at the edges of the diaphragmatic perforations in many cases of CPX [22]; these findings may support the migration theory in the etiopathology of catamenial pneumothorax.

4. Clinical manifestations and diagnosis

The typical clinical manifestations of CPX include spontaneous pneumothorax with or before menses presented with pain, dyspnea, and cough. Scapular and thoracic pain may also be present before or during menstruation. There may also be a history of previous episodes of spontaneous pneumothorax, history of previous uterine surgery, primary or secondary infertility or uterine scratching, pelvic endometriosis diagnosis, and history of catamenial hemoptysis or catamenial hemothorax [30].

Medical history and occurrence of typical symptoms are crucial for the diagnosis of catamenial pneumothorax, and these findings should be systematically investigated [11]. Although existence of these findings creates high suspicion on catamenial pneumothorax, their absence does not exclude a diagnosis of catamenial pneumothorax [24, 30].

Intermittent presentations out of menstrual bleeding time should not exclude the diagnosis of noncatamenial endometriosis-associated pneumothorax even in the absence of symptoms and pelvic endometriosis [9, 24, 38].

The clinical course of CPX is usually mild or moderate, but sometimes be life-threatening. Widespread thoracic endometriosis after previous operations is reported in the literature as case reports [39]. A young woman who experienced an episode of life-threatening hemopneumothorax who has been treated by urgent tube thoracostomy and thoracotomy was reported by Morcos et al. [39]. Lung wedge resection, parietal pleurectomy, and partial diaphragmatic excision have also been performed in this case.

Patients with CPX are reported to have a mean age of 35 (range 15–54) years at presentation [40].

Catamenial pneumothorax can also have very rare presentations in the literature. Simultaneous occurrence of pneumoperitoneum and catamenial pneumothorax [33, 34], catamenial pneumoperitoneum mimicking acute abdomen in a woman with multiple episodes of pneumothorax [35], pneumothorax, and pneumoperitoneum in a patient with spontaneous diaphragmatic rupture has been reported in the literature [41].

Medical history is the main pathway on the way to the diagnosis of CPX. Synchronicity of the clinical course with menses is the main character of the disease, but on the other hand intraoperative visual inspection and appropriate histological examination of the pathognomonic lesions are crucial for the diagnosis of endometriosis-related pneumothorax. The surgeon needs to be vigilant because it can easily be missed if not cautious [7, 24, 29, 42].

5. Imaging diagnostic criteria

Chest radiogram, computed tomography, and magnetic resonance imaging are the imaging modalities that can be used for the diagnosis of catamenial pneumothorax. Although there are no disease-specific diagnostic criteria, pneumothorax is usually right sided. On the other hand, left-sided or bilateral cases are present. Air-fluid leveling may also occur at chest radiogram, in some cases. Hemopneumothorax may also be a part of clinical course [24, 30]. Loculated fluids can be seen in cases with the history of previous surgery [39].

Only in a few number of cases, small diaphragmatic defects can be detected with careful examination of chest radiogram, which refers to diaphragmatic perforations. Also when a right-sided pneumothorax with a round opacity on the right hemidiaphragm occurs, liver protrusion into a large diaphragm defect is suspected [21, 43]. This type of partial intrathoracic liver herniation at the right hemidiaphragm on chest radiogram and CT [24, 44] has been reported in the literature. There are also reports in the literature regarding diaphragmatic masses on CT [23] and pleural masses on MRI that refers to endometrial implants [45].

CT findings of hemoptysis are nonspecific; they may differ from a focal ground-glass opacity to consolidation because of alveolar filling, similarly in hemoptysis caused by other disease [46]. Especially in nondependent lung parenchyma, these findings facilitate the location of the site of bleeding. In the early period of the disease, endobronchial clots may be present, which cause atelectasis in some cases. There are also reports revealing band-like opacities referring to linear fibrosis sites, which result from chronic hemorrhage [46].

MRI is another imaging modality that can be used for confirming thoracic endometriosis in some cases. CT has some disadvantages especially in spatial resolution, but MRI has high-contrast resolution and can better characterize hemorrhagic lesions. Representation of diaphragmatic or pleural implants with MRI can help to clarify the diagnosis and management of the patient with catamenial pneumothorax [46].

MRI may also be useful for patients with catamenial hydropneumothorax; small pleural endometriomas characterized by the presence of small cystic hyperintense lesions can be revealed by MRI images of visceral or parietal pleura [46].

Coexisting pneumothorax and pneumoperitoneum are other findings that can be seen on radiography and computed tomography [33, 34].

6. Tumor antigens

Increased levels of cancer antigen 125 have been associated with endometriosis. It is not considered a specific marker, but it can play a role in early diagnosis of endometriosis-related pneumothorax [47, 48].

7. Characteristic findings of catamenial pneumothorax

Characteristic lesions of the catamenial pneumothorax include single or multiple diaphragmatic spots, perforations, nodules, and visceral or parietal pleural spots and nodules. Pericardial nodules have also been reported in some cases.

These lesions have not been found in all patients with catamenial pneumothorax, but they have been revealed in some cases with noncatamenial pneumothorax. Detection of endometrial tissue is not mandatory in these lesions. On the other hand, endometrial tissue has usually been found in diaphragmatic and pleural nodules, but it is rarely detected at the edges of the diaphragmatic perforations [30].

Visceral and parietal pleural lesions are less frequently detected than diaphragmatic defects, spots, and nodules.

7.1 Diaphragmatic lesions

The diaphragmatic lesions usually located at the centrum tendineum and can be single or multiple. They usually settle adjacent to nodules. They can be outlined as perforations, fenestrations, holes, stomata, and pores [24, 30, 49] (**Figure 1a** and **b**).

They can be tiny holes measuring 1–3 millimeters in diameter [7, 50], or larger defects measuring up to 10 mm [4, 18] or more than 10 mm [8] or represent as undetected holes proven only by diagnostic pneumoperitoneum [42].

Diaphragmatic defects are usually found close to coexisting nodules or spots, and endometrial tissue is sporadically found at the edges of the defects [4, 9, 11, 22]. This situation supports the theory claiming that the diaphragmatic defects represent the breakdown of endometrial implants during menstrual cycle [22, 24].

There are also case reports of larger lacerations that accompany with intrathoracic liver protrusion, but these presentations are very rare.

A patient with catamenial pneumothorax on the right hemithorax was reported by Pryshchepau et al. Liver of the patient was protruded through a large diaphragmatic defect [44].

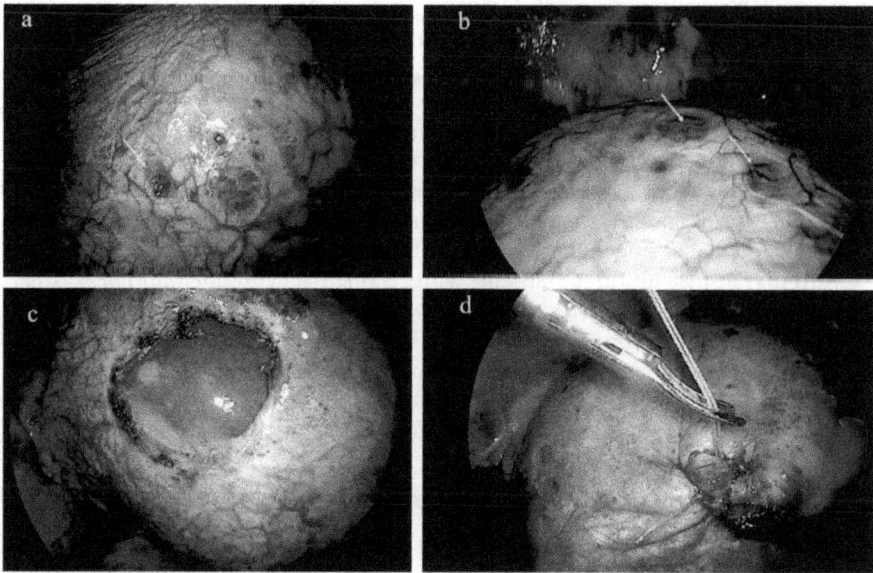

Figure 1.
(a) and (b) Thoracoscopic view of diaphragmatic endometriosis. Fenestrations can be seen on the surface of the diaphragm (arrows). (c) The liver is visible after surgical resection. (d) Sutured diaphragm after endometriosis resection. Images are used with the permission of Demetrio Larrain [49].

Visouli et al. also reported five cases of catamenial pneumothorax [24], which contains a case very similar regarding liver protrusion, and they have recommended that these findings should be included in the characteristic findings of catamenial and thoracic endometriosis-related pneumothorax, although this presentation is very rare [24].

Catamenial pneumothorax with a huge diaphragmatic laceration and partial intrathoracic liver herniation was reported by Bobbio et al. [43], and Makhija et al. [51] reported a patient with multiple diaphragmatic fenestrations. The largest lesion was reported to have a diameter of 10 cm.

Spontaneous rupture of the right hemidiaphragm and intrathoracic liver herniation was also reported in the literature [41]. Pneumothorax and pneumoperitoneum was detected in a patient with a history of premenstrual periscapular pain. At the edge of the diaphragmatic defect, a nodule looking like an endometrial implant was found in that patient. Histological examination of the nodule revealed endometriosis with hemosiderin-loaded macrophages. This case is considered as endometriosis-related, but the histological criteria set by the authors was not appropriate [9, 11]. Additionally, previously mentioned cases of large diaphragmatic defects were considered to be limited diaphragmatic ruptures and stated that endometriosis was responsible for these ruptures [43, 44].

7.2 Thoracic lesions

Endometrial tissue is usually detected on histopathological examination of the spots or nodules accompanying catamenial pneumothorax so these lesions are considered to be endometrial implants. Diaphragm, visceral, and parietal pleura are the common sites for location. Pericardial implants were also reported by Fonseca et al. [52]. The lesions may be single or multiple and may have varying size. They may have different presentations in color as brown, purple, red, violet, blueberry, black, white, grayish, and grayish-purple [1–20, 51].

Diaphragmatic and thoracic lesions may be present in all cases, but on the other hand, only one or more of them can be seen either [1–21, 39, 53, 54].

In some cases of catamenial pneumothorax, characteristic findings may be absent and blebs and bullae may be the only pathological findings. In some cases, no characteristic thoracic findings may be detected [7, 12, 20, 22–24].

Detection of characteristic lesions during thoracotomy or thoracoscopy depends on thorough and deliberate examination of the thorax, including the diaphragm. This also depends on the stage of the disease and catamenial behavior of the disease and longer-term variation [22, 24, 30, 42].

8. Surgical treatment of catamenial pneumothorax

Surgical treatment is the gold standard in treatment of catamenial pneumo-thorax, not only for its better results but less recurrences after treatment as well. Surgery has better results compared with medical treatment [1–20].

Korom et al. [7] reviewed 195 cases of CPX among 229 cases and reported that 154 cases (78%) were treated surgically. Among surgically treated patients, diaphragmatic repair (38%), pleurodesis (81%), and lung wedge resection (20%) were performed.

There is common consensus in the literature that the appropriate approach to CPX has to be minimally invasive so video-assisted thoracoscopic surgery (VATS) is the choice of treatment. VATS not only provides magnification but complete visualization of diaphragm as well [23].

Video-assisted thoracoscopic surgery (VATS) has been mainly in use since 2000 in the treatment of thoracic diseases with several advantages over conven-tional thoracotomy. Incision may be extended when extensive diaphragmatic repair is required, and also a muscle-sparing thoracotomy may offer better access in such cases. Thoracotomy may be an option especially in recurrent interventions or in reoperations [4–28, 30].

The lung examination for bullae, bleb, and air leakage is very important, but the diaphragm should also be carefully examined for fenestrations and spots or nod-ules. In addition, it is critical to examine the parietal pleura, lung, and pericardium in terms of spots and nodules.

Bagan et al. recommended the use of surgical treatment during menstrua-tion. Thus, they stated that endometriotic lesions may be better visualized during menstrual period [22]. Slasky et al. used the pneumoperitoneum method to reveal unseen diaphragmatic fenestrations [42]. Identification of the lesions within the thorax is made easier by the magnification provided by VATS [4–28, 30]. The tissue samples from these lesions make it easy to diagnose thoracic endometriosis [10].

Resection of all visible lesions such as bullae or bleb and also resection of endometriosis-induced thoracic lesions have been recommended by Alifano et al. Limited wedge resection of the diseased lung tissue, limited parietal pleurectomy, and partial diaphragmatic resection were suggested surgical techniques for the elimination of intrathoracic lesions [4].

Excision and wedge resection of bullae and blebs [7, 12, 23, 30], along with pleurodesis or pleurectomy, has been mainly performed in the literature [7, 8, 12, 23, 30, 47]. Pleurodesis was found to be the most common intervention [29]. The majority of pleurodesis performed was mechanical pleurodesis (abrasion or pleu-rectomy), which has been found to be more successful in comparison to chemical pleurodesis [6].

Addressing the diaphragmatic pathology is of paramount importance. Diaphragmatic plication and/or resection of the diseased area have been reported [7, 12, 23, 24, 30, 49] (**Figure 1c and d**).

Recurrence is the most common complication of CPX, and there are reported recurrence rates of 20–40% [4, 7, 41, 51]. Alifano et al. suggested that diaphragmatic resection with removal of endometrial implants is the preferred method compared to single diaphragmatic plication because plication has an disadvantage of leaving endometrial implants untreated [29, 38]. Still, recurrences may develop even after diaphragmatic resection [29].

Fewer recurrences after diaphragmatic coverage with a polyglactin mesh were reported by Bagan et al. To prevent recurrences, they suggested a systematic diaphragmatic covering, including the normal appearance of diaphragms, treating ocular defects, strengthening the diaphragm, and inducing adhesions to the lung [7].

There are also reports on diaphragmatic coverage with a polyglactin or polypropylene mesh [8], a polytetrafluoroethylene (PTFE) mesh [15], or a bovine pericardial patch [24], which has been reported with good mid-term results.

9. Medical treatment

Hormonal treatment has a supplementary role in the treatment of catamenial pneumothorax. With the administration of hormonal therapy, it is possible to prevent recurrences of catamenial pneumothorax.

A multidisciplinary approach is mandatory for the management of the disease and administration of gonadotrophin-releasing hormone (GnRH) analogue, which results in the lack of menses, and is suggested for all patients with proven catamenial pneumothorax in the early postoperative period for 6–12 months [4, 7, 8, 22, 24, 30, 48]. Patients without documented catamenial character or histologically proven thoracic endometriosis may also benefit from hormonal treatment even in the presence of characteristic lesions [24, 30].

Woman's plans concerning pregnancy are very crucial, when deciding whether to start hormonal therapy or not. In such therapies, oral contraceptive pills (estrogen-progestogen) are usually used which induce menses every 28 days or they are used continuously without inducing menses. These pills also include progestogens, and they may be administered orally, intramuscularly, or in intrauterine way.

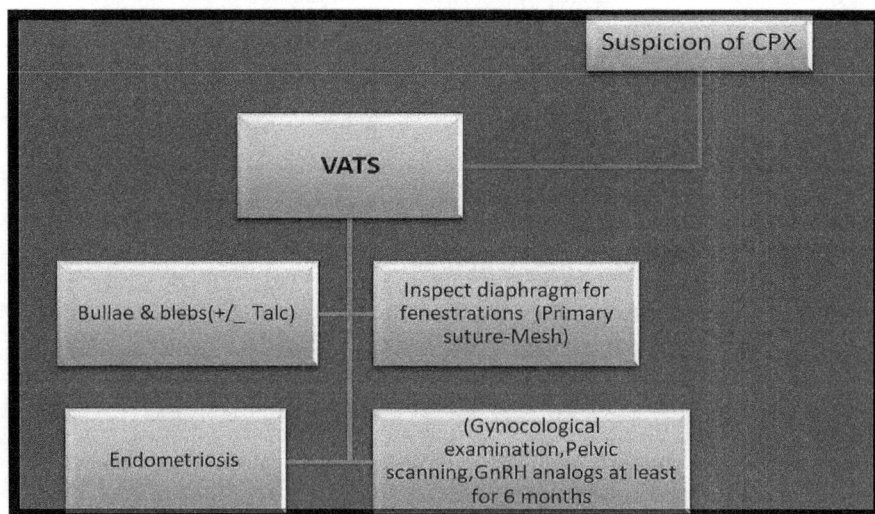

Figure 2.
Accepted surgical algorithm and treatment in catamenial pneumothorax.

There are also several medications, which are currently in use. Medical treatment is recommended in patients when catamenial pneumothorax is associated with endometriosis [17].

The aim of early GnRH analogue delivery is to prevent cyclic hormonal changes and to suppress the activity of the ectopic endometrium until effective pleurodesis occurs, because time is needed for the formation of effective pleural adhesions [38].

Hormonal treatment is advised for longer periods especially after reoperations for catamenial pneumothorax.

Proven ineffectiveness of the therapy or significant side effects of the drugs are the contraindications of hormonal therapy [29].

There is an accepted surgical algorithm and treatment in catamenial pneumothorax [55], which is described in **Figure 2** in detail.

10. Results of treatment

Practically, surgery for catamenial pneumothorax has very low mortality and morbidity. Recurrence is the most common complication of CPX, and there are reported recurrence rates of 20–40% [4, 7, 41, 53].

High recurrence rates are much higher than surgically treated idiopathic pneumothorax [8–10, 22–24, 29].

A low recurrence rate (8.3%), at a mean follow-up of 45.8 months, was reported by Attaran et al., by video thoracoscopic abrasion and pleurectomy, diaphragmatic repair and PTFE mesh coverage for the repair of diaphragmatic defects, and a routine postoperative hormonal treatment [55].

Also Alifano et al. reported that the highest postoperative recurrence rate in 114 women who were operated due to recurrent spontaneous pneumothorax was in the catamenial pneumothorax group (32%), and this was followed by a noncatamenial endometriosis-associated pneumothorax group (27%). They also reported a recurrence rate of 5.3%, at a mean of 32.7 months of follow-up, in patients with noncatamenial nonendometriosis-associated pneumothorax [32].

Incomplete surgical treatment of lesions and lack of additional hormonal treatment in the early postoperative period [23, 24, 38–54] may increase the risk of recurrence [24, 30, 38–56].

11. Conclusions

Young women with pneumothorax, especially in the perimenstrual period, should be suspected of catamenial pneumothorax. Failure occurs most frequently when recurrent catamenial pneumothorax occurs.

The lesions of the parietal and visceral pleura should be carefully examined and removed during surgery. Diaphragm reconstruction is required every time when fenestrations are detected in diaphragm.

Hormonal therapy is also recommended because it facilitates the effectiveness of the surgical results.

Multidisciplinary approach with early postoperative hormonal treatment, which deals with all thoracic pathologies including disease awareness, early diagnosis, diaphragmatic repair, and surgical management of the main chronic systemic disease, may eventually lead to a reduction in the rate of recurrence of catamenial pneumothorax [3–13, 15, 23, 24, 30, 32].

Treatment of women of childbearing age is different from men of the same age group. CPX should be excluded in the cohort of women, especially when the pneumothorax is repeated. Full examination of the diaphragm should be part of the operation. Surgeons who perform VATS should be experienced to resect and repair diaphragms with fenestrations and endometrial deposits, including keyhole laying down of synthetic mesh.

Conflict of interest

There is no conflict of interest.

Thanks

We would like to thank Dr. Demetrio Larraín who kindly gave us permission to use his images in our chapter.

Author details

Sezai Celik[1]* and Ezel Erşen[2]

1 Department of Thoracic Surgery, Avicenna Hospitals, Istanbul, Turkey

2 Cerrahpasa Medical Faculty, Department of Thoracic Surgery, Istanbul University - Cerrahpasa, Istanbul, Turkey

*Address all correspondence to: siyamie@gmail.com

IntechOpen

References

[1] Maurer ER, Schaal JA, Mendez FL Jr. Chronic recurring spontaneous pneumothorax due to endometriosis of the diaphragm. JAMA. 1958;**168**:2013-2014

[2] Lillington GA, Mitchell SP, Wood GA. Catamenial pneumothorax. JAMA. 1972;**219**:1328-1332

[3] Joseph J, Sahn SA. Thoracic endometriosis syndrome: New observations from an analysis of 110 cases. The American Journal of Medicine. 1996;**100**:164-170

[4] Alifano M, Roth T, Broët SC, Schussler O, Magdeleinat P, Regnard J-F. Catamenial pneumothorax: A prospective study. Chest. 2003;**124**:1004-1008

[5] Azizad-Pinto P, Clarke D. Thoracic endometriosis syndrome: Case report and review of the literature. The Permanente Journal. 2014;**18**:61-65

[6] Bricelj K, Srpčič M, Ražem A, Snoj Ž. Catamenial pneumothorax since introduction of video-assisted thoracoscopic surgery. Wiener Klinische Wochenschrift. 2017;**129**(19-20):717-726

[7] Korom S, Canyurt H, Missbach A, Schneiter D, Kurrer MO, Haller U, et al. Catamenial pneumothorax revisited: Clinical approach and systematic review of the literature. The Journal of Thoracic and Cardiovascular Surgery. 2004;**128**:502-508

[8] Leong AC, Coonar AS, Lang-Lazdunski L. Catamenial pneumothorax: Surgical repair of the diaphragm and hormone treatment. Annals of the Royal College of Surgeons of England. 2006;**88**:547-549

[9] Alifano M, Jablonski C, Kadiri H, Falcoz P, Gompel A, Camilleri-Broet S, et al. Catamenial and noncatamenial, endometriosis-related or nonendometriosis-related pneumothorax referred for surgery. American Journal of Respiratory and Critical Care Medicine. 2007;**176**:1048-1053

[10] Alifano M. Catamenial pneumothorax. Current Opinion in Pulmonary Medicine. 2010;**16**:381-386

[11] Rousset-Jablonski C, Alifano M, Plu-Bureau G, Camilleri-Broet S, Rousset P, Regnard J-F, et al. Catamenialpneumothorax and endometriosis-related pneumothorax: Clinical features and risk factors. Human Reproduction. 2011;**26**(9): 2322-2329. DOI: 10.1093/humrep/der189

[12] Marshall MB, Ahmed Z, Kucharczuk JC, Kaiser LR, Shrager JB. Catamenial pneumothorax: Optimal hormonal and surgical management. European Journal of Cardio-Thoracic Surgery. 2005;**27**:662-666

[13] Thomas V, Thomas E, Lionel J. Catamenial pneumothorax: A rare phenomenon? The Journal of Obstetrics and Gynecology of India. 2013;**63**(6):424-425

[14] Rousset-Jablonski C, Alifano M, Plu-Bureau G, Camilleri-Broet S, Rousset P, Regnard JF, et al. Catamenial pneumothorax endometriosis-related pneumothorax: Clinical features and risk factors. Human Reproduction. 2011;**26**:2322-2329

[15] Attaran S, Bille A, Karenovics W, Lang-Lazdunski L. Videothoracoscopic repair of diaphragm and pleurectomy/abrasion in patients with catamenial pneumothorax: A 9-year experience. Chest. 2013;**143**:1066-1069

[16] Channabasavaiah AD, Joseph JV. Thoracic endometriosis: Revisiting

the association between clinical presentation and thoracic pathology based on thoracoscopic findings in 110 patients. Medicine (Baltimore). 2010;**89**:183-188

[17] Marjański T, Sowa K, Czapla A, Rzyman W. Catamenial pneumothorax—A review of the literature. Kardiochirurgia i Torakochirurgia Polska. 2016;**13**:117-121

[18] Cowl CT, Dunn WF, Deschamps C. Visualisations of diaphragmatic fenestration associated with catamenial pneumothorax. The Annals of Thoracic Surgery. 1999;**68**:1413-1414

[19] Haga T, Kurihara M, Kataoka H, Ebana H. Clinical-pathological findings of catamenial pneumothorax: Comparison between recurrent cases and nonrecurrent cases. Annals of Thoracic and Cardiovascular Surgery. 2014;**20**:202-206

[20] Majak P, Langebrekke A, Hagen OM, Qviqstad E. Catamenial pneumothorax, clinical manifestations—A multidisciplinary challenge. Pneumonologia i Alergologia Polska. 2011;**79**:347-350

[21] Roth T, Alifano M, Schussler O, Magdaleinat P, Regnard JF. Catamenial pneumothorax: Chest X-ray sign and thoracoscopic treatment. The Annals of Thoracic Surgery. 2002;**74**:563-565

[22] Bagan P, Le Pimpec Barthes F, Assouad J, et al. Catamenial pneumothorax: Retrospective study of surgical treatment. The Annals of Thoracic Surgery. 2003;**75**:378-381

[23] Ciriaco P, Negri G, Libretti L, et al. Surgical treatment of catamenial pneumothorax: A single centre experience. Interactive Cardiovascular and Thoracic Surgery. 2009;**8**:349-352

[24] Visouli AN, Darwiche K, Mpakas A, et al. Catamenial pneumothorax: A rare entity? Report of 5 cases and review of the literature. Journal of Thoracic Disease. 2012;**4**:17-31

[25] Schoenfeld A, Ziv E, Zeelel Y, et al. Catamenial pneumothorax—A literature review and report of an unusual case. Obstetrical & Gynecological Survey. 1986;**41**:20-24

[26] Blanco S, Hernando F, Gómez A, et al. Catamenial pneumothorax caused by diaphragmatic endometriosis. The Journal of Thoracic and Cardiovascular Surgery. 1998;**116**:179-180

[27] Nakamura H, Konishiike J, Sugamura A, et al. Epidemiology of spontaneous pneumothorax in women. Chest. 1986;**89**:378-382

[28] Shearin RP, Hepper NG, Payne WS. Recurrent spontaneous pneumothorax concurrent with menses. Mayo Clinic Proceedings. 1974;**49**:98-101

[29] Alifano M, Legras A, Rousset-Jablonski C, et al. Pneumothorax recurrence after surgery in women: Clinicopathologic characteristics and management. The Annals of Thoracic Surgery. 2011;**92**:322-326

[30] Visouli AN, Zarogoulidis K, Kougioumtzi I, et al. Catamenial pneumothorax. Journal of Thoracic Disease. 2014;**6**:S448-S460

[31] Laws HL, Fox LS, Younger JB. Bilateral catamenial pneumothorax. Archives of Surgery. 1977;**112**:627-628

[32] Van Schil PE, Vercauteren SR, Vermeire PA, et al. Catamenial pneumothorax caused by thoracic endometriosis. The Annals of Thoracic Surgery. 1996;**62**:585-586

[33] Downey DB, Towers MJ, Poon PY, et al. Pneumoperitoneum with catamenial pneumothorax. AJR. American Journal of Roentgenology. 1990;**155**:29-30

[34] Jablonski C, Alifano M, Regnard JF, et al. Pneumoperitoneum associated with catamenial pneumothorax in women with thoracic endometriosis. Fertility and Sterility. 2009;**91**:930. e19-930.e22

[35] Grunewald RA, Wiggins J. Pulmonary endometriosis mimicking acute abdomen. Postgraduate Medical Journal. 1988;**64**:865-866

[36] Nezhat C, King LP, Paka C, et al. Bilateral thoracic endometriosis affecting the lung and diaphragm. JSLS. 2012;**16**:140-142

[37] Andrade-Alegre R, González W. Catamenial pneumothorax. Journal of the American College of Surgeons. 2007;**205**:724

[38] Alifano M, Magdeleinat P, Regnard JF. Catamenial pneumothorax: Some commentaries. The Journal of Thoracic and Cardiovascular Surgery. 2005;**129**:1199

[39] Morcos M, Alifano M, Gompel A, et al. Life-threatening endometriosis-related hemopneumothorax. The Annals of Thoracic Surgery. 2006;**82**:726-729

[40] Suwatanapongched T, Boonsarngsuk V, Amornputtisathaporn N, Leelachaikul P. Thoracic endometriosis with catamenial haemoptysis and pneumothorax: Computed tomography findings and long-term follow-up after danazol treatment. Singapore Medical Journal. 2015;**56**:e120-e123

[41] Triponez F, Alifano M, Bobbio A, et al. Endometriosis-related spontaneous diaphragmatic rupture. Interactive Cardiovascular and Thoracic Surgery. 2010;**11**:485-487

[42] Slasky BS, Siewers RD, Lecky JW, et al. Catamenial pneumothorax: The roles of diaphragmatic defects and endometriosis. AJR. American Journal of Roentgenology. 1982;**138**:639-643

[43] Bobbio A, Carbognani P, Ampollini L, et al. Diaphragmatic laceration, partial liver herniation and catamenial pneumothorax. Asian Cardiovascular & Thoracic Annals. 2007;**15**:249-251

[44] Pryshchepau M, Gossot D, Magdeleinat P. Unusual presentation of catamenial pneumothorax. European Journal of Cardio-Thoracic Surgery. 2010;**37**:1221

[45] Picozzi G, Beccani D, Innocenti F, et al. MRI features of pleural endometriosis after catamenial haemothorax. Thorax. 2007;**62**:744

[46] Rousset P, Rousset-Jablonski C, Alifano M, Mansuet-Lupo A, Buy JN, Revel MP. Thoracic endometriosis syndrome: CT and MRI features. Clinical Radiology. 2014;**69**(3):323-330

[47] Attaran M, Falcone T, Goldberg J. Endometriosis: Still tough to diagnose and treat. Cleveland Clinic Journal of Medicine. 2002;**69**:647-653

[48] Hagneré P, Deswarte S, Leleu O. Thoracic endometriosis: A difficult diagnosis. Revue des Maladies Respiratoires. 2011;**28**:908-912

[49] Larraín D, Suárez F, Braun H, Chapochnick J, Diaz L, Rojas I. Thoracic and diaphragmatic endometriosis: Single-institution experience using novel, broadened diagnostic criteria. Journal of the Turkish-German Gynecological Association. 2018;**19**:116-121

[50] Suzuki S, Yasuda K, Matsumura Y, et al. Left-side catamenial pneumothorax with endometrial tissue on the visceral pleura. The Japanese Journal of Thoracic and Cardiovascular Surgery. 2006;**54**:225-227

[51] Makhija Z, Marrinan M. A case of Catamenial pneumothorax with diaphragmatic fenestrations. The Journal of Emergency Medicine. 2012;**43**:e1-e3

[52] Fonseca P. Catamenial pneumothorax: A multifactorial etiology. The Journal of Thoracic and Cardiovascular Surgery. 1998;**116**:872-873

[53] Kumakiri J, Kumakiri Y, Miyamoto H, et al. Gynecologic evaluation of catamenial pneumothorax associated with endometriosis. Journal of Minimally Invasive Gynecology. 2010;**17**:593-599

[54] Kronauer CM. Images in clinical medicine. Catamenial pneumothorax. The New England Journal of Medicine. 2006;**355**:e9

[55] Baysungur V, Tezel C, Okur E, Yilmaz B. Recurrent pneumothorax diagnosed as catamenial after videothoracoscopic examination of the pleural cavity. Surgical Laparoscopy, Endoscopy & Percutaneous Techniques. 2011;**21**:e81-ee3

[56] Mikroulis DA, Didilis VN, Konstantinou F, et al. Catamenial pneumothorax. The Thoracic and Cardiovascular Surgeon. 2008;**56**:374-375

Chapter 5

Controversies in Pneumothorax Treatment

Khalid Amer

Abstract

Surgical intervention either by video-assisted thoracoscopic surgery (VATS) or open procedure proved its worth in reducing the incidence of recurrence in pneumothorax. However, many controversies surround the management of this common medical condition. Despite advances in knowledge and technology, chest physicians and surgeons could not be more divisive about the management of pneumothorax. There are no two thoracic surgical centres and possibly no two surgeons within the same hospital that agree on the management of the different aspects of pneumothorax. The variability in reported outcomes and the paucity of published multicentre randomised controlled trials (RCT) highlight the need for further studies investigating the best options for pneumostasis and pleurodesis. This chapter aims at discussing some of these controversies and reviews the literature at its current state of evidence.

Keywords: pneumothorax, video-assisted thoracic surgery, thoracotomy, pleurodesis, air leak, surgical emphysema, intercostal drain, COPD

1. Introduction

The Red Indians knew that the North American buffalo had a single pleural cavity. A single arrow to the chest was enough to collapse both lungs and expedite the death of the beast. On the other hand, the elephant is unique insofar as it is the only mammal whose pleural space is obliterated by connective tissue. This natural pleurodesis has been known for over 300 years but only recently explained [1]. Apparently, the elephant is the only mammal that can remain submerged far below the surface of the water while snorkelling. It is intriguing though that the foetal elephant has normal pleural spaces that obliterate later in gestation [2]. Humans are slightly luckier; they enjoy two pleural spaces separated by mediastinal structures; if one lung collapses, the other one sustains life. However, there are reports in the literature of some patients with pleuro-pleural congenital communications, presenting with simultaneous bilateral pneumothoraces, the so-called buffalo chest [3].

Humans collapse their lungs frequently, and the different ways we deal with this common condition match its frequency. There is bound to be differences in opinion, and the multicentre randomised controlled trials (RCT) have not come up with a solid protocol to guide management. There was no general agreement on therapy when Ruckley and McCormac of the Royal Infirmary of Edinburgh described the management of pneumothorax in 1966 [4]. There is no agreement at our present time still, despite the technological advances in our knowledge and the available randomised controlled trials. We could not agree more with Robert Cerfolio et al. on their statement that "although thoracic surgeons are the best trained physicians to manage chest tubes and pleural problems, they often do not speak the same language or recommend similar treatment algorithms even to each other" [5].

2. The physiology of respiration and pneumothorax

The pressure in the pleural space is determined by the difference between the lung elastic recoil and volume changes of the semi-rigid chest wall. The rib cage moves in three dimensions; the girdle handle movement of the ribs increases the anteroposterior and the lateral dimensions of the chest, whereas the piston-pump movement of the diaphragm leads to an increase in the vertical dimension of the chest cavity. The chest and diaphragm movements create a physiological negative pressure within the pleural space that forces the lung to change shape and volume with the respiratory cycle, resulting in inflation and deflation. Neutralising this negative pressure in the pleural space leads to lung collapse, as the elastic structure of the lung favours its collapse (recoil). Pneumothorax or air in the pleural space invariably leads to lung collapse. A thin film of fluid exists between the parietal and visceral pleurae to lubricate the sliding of these two structures, roughly 15 mls in a 70 kg adult person. The fluid is a microvascular filtrate produced by the parietal pleura and is cleared also by the parietal pleural lymphatics, a process similar to that in any other body organ.

3. Epidemiology and pathology of pneumothorax

The term "pneumothorax" was first coined by Itard (1803), but it was Laennec (1819) who described its clinical picture [6]. The term refers to "air in the pleural space". Pneumothorax is a significant global health problem ranking high on the list of common medical conditions, especially in the emergency department. In the United Kingdom (UK), the overall person consulting rate for pneumothorax (primary and secondary combined) was 24 per 100,000 each year for men and 9.8 per 100,000 each year for women. Hospital admissions for pneumothorax as a primary diagnosis occurred at an overall incidence of 16.7 per 100,000 per year for men and 5.8 per 100,000 per year for women. Mortality rates were 1.26 per million per year for men and 0.62 per million per year for women [7].

How does air gain access to the pleural space? Well, there are several mechanisms for this to happen. Communication between atmospheric air and the pleural space can result from trauma, penetrating injuries, impalements, stabs, bullets and ammunition. Fractured ribs puncturing the lung is a common cause for traumatic pneumothorax, recorded in our accident and emergency department (58 patients between January 2007 and 2018). Pneumothorax could also occur spontaneously and unprovoked due to a puncture in the visceral pleura, allowing air to pass from the open alveoli or small bronchi directly into the pleural space. Air can gain access to the pleural space from holes or tears in the aero-digestive system, such as neck stabs to the trachea, or a bronchopleural fistula due to tuberculosis or oesophageal rupture. Iatrogenic pneumothorax is caused by interventional procedures such as central line access, bronchoscopy, oesophagoscopy, insertion of stents, etc. Air in the peritoneal cavity can gain access to the chest through holes (fenestrations) in the diaphragm. This is one of the explanations of catamenial pneumothorax [8, 9]. Pneumothorax following substance abuse and recreational drugs, especially cocaine, cannabis and marijuana, has been associated with bullous disease and pneumothorax. However, many is the time bullae are absent and the pneumothorax is associated with pneumomediastinum or pneumopericardium. In these instances, air leak does not track to the lung surface, but instead it tracks into the connective tissue separating the lung segments and heads towards the hilum. To be comprehensive one should not forget about gas producing organisms which might generate air in the pleural space without any of the above breaches.

One-way valve motion of air from the lung to pleural space is a dreaded complication. It could lead to life-threatening tension pneumothorax. In this complication, not only the ipsilateral lung collapses, but the mounting pressure on the mediastinum pushes the central structures and restricts movement of the contralateral lung. Dislocation of the heart to the contralateral side might reach a critical degree that kinks the vena cavae and severely restricts venous return to the heart. This could result in hyperacute heart failure and death [10]. Cyanosis, sweating, severe tachypnoea, tachycardia and hypotension may indicate the presence of this medical emergency. Diagnosis of tension pneumothorax is clinical, and a needle or chest drain must be inserted, before obtaining a chest X-ray.

4. Classification and treatment

Eighty percent of pneumothoraces are secondary to trauma, and 20% spontaneous without provocation. Two big categories of spontaneous pneumothorax (SP) exist, with bimodal age distribution: primary SP 15–35 years of age and secondary SP +55 years of age. Pneumothorax is distinctly rare among children less than 15 years. Wilcox et al. reported 17 cases in 12 years [11]. Primary SP occurs on a background of normal lungs, whereas secondary SP is associated with diseased lungs, such as emphysema, chronic obstructive pulmonary disease (COPD), lung fibrosis and cystic fibrosis. Secondary SP is strongly related to cigarette smoking and associated with a higher morbidity and mortality compared to primary SP. Primary pneumothorax has been associated with rupture of apical bullae or blebs (**Figure 1**) and has a 54.2% chance of recurring after the first episode [12]. In the UK the male-to-female ratio is 3:1 [7].

The British Thoracic Society (BTS) has published an updated summary of the management of pneumothorax in 2010 [10]. Similar guidelines were published earlier by the American College of Physicians in 2001 [13] and later by the European Task Force in 2015 [14]. Breathlessness and the size of pneumothorax influence the management of SP. There is a general consensus that conservative management should be tried in the first episode, as conservative management of small pneumothoraces has been shown to be safe [10, 15]. Surgery proved that recurrence is less, and video-assisted

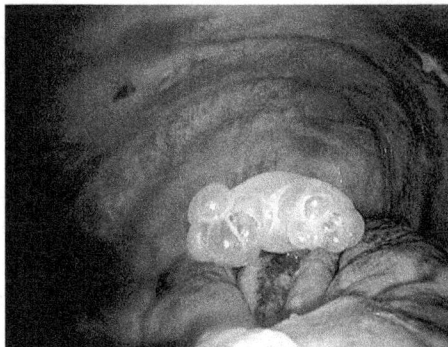

Figure 1.
Single apical bulla, a common cause of primary spontaneous pneumothorax.

thoracoscopic surgery (VATS) has opened the option of treating even the first-time pneumothorax on semi-urgent basis [16–18]. However, there has been no general agreement on the most effective type of surgery or that which is most accepted by patients. Ostensibly such a choice should result in the least incidence of recurrence. Axillary thoracotomy, full posterolateral thoracotomy, limited lateral muscle sparing mini-thoracotomy and triportal, biportal and needlescopic uniportal VATS have all been utilised [10, 18, 19]. A subxiphoid approach has also been tried and reported [20]. These operations have two objectives: firstly, to deal with the source of air leak (pneumostasis) by bullectomy/blebectomy, etc. and, secondly, to obliterate the pleural space leading to permanent adherence of the lung to the chest wall (pleurodesis or symphysis). In essence, we strive to emulate the elephant pleural space and prevent recurrence.

In the 1950s and 1960s, the treatment varied from extremely conservative bed rest only to early insertion of a Malecot catheter through the second intercostal space anteriorly (very painful!) and thoracotomy or bilateral thoracotomies for non-resolving cases [4]. Today's management is nowhere near that, and minimal access surgery or VATS has taken up the management of pneumothorax to a new level [19].

Several randomised and non-randomised trials (RCT) looked into the difference between the optimal surgical techniques in SP [21]. There is no evidence to support the superiority of either VATS or open thoracotomy in the treatment of pneumothorax because the number of randomised trials is sparse and they are underpowered to detect any meaningful difference. Barker et al. published an important meta-analysis of four randomised and 25 non-randomised studies performed in 2007 comparing VATS to open thoracotomy [22]. Complex statistical tests of homogeneity and sensitivity analysis with a hypothetical model biased against open surgery were undertaken. RCT without comparative control groups were excluded. They reported a worrying fourfold increase in the recurrence of pneumothorax following VATS procedure compared to thoracotomy. Their relative risk (RR) favours open surgery; however, postoperative pain could not be assessed since most studies did not report this outcome. Neither did they report on length of hospital stay, due to severe heterogeneity in reporting. A similar previous study by Sedrakyan et al. looking only at the randomised trials did not show this difference [23]. The conclusion is that recurrence following VATS averaged 4.5%, whereas that following mini-thoracotomy was 2.3%. Waller et al. randomised 30 patients to VATS and 30 to open thoracotomy [24]. They concluded that VATS is superior to thoracotomy in the treatment of primary SP but had a higher recurrence rate in secondary SP. Ayed et al. in a randomised trial found VATS superior to thoracotomy but reported higher recurrence rates [25]. A best evidence topic by Vohra et al. reiterated on the superiority of VATS insofar as pain control, less hospital stay and better early lung functions [26]. It stopped short of recommending open thoracotomy for the treatment of this condition, quoting the Barker study. It is hard to imagine that any contemporary surgeon or clinician would recommend open thoracotomy over VATS to their patients, based on this evidence. VATS is the most favoured approach by patients. The Barker study, despite their extensive heterogeneity tests, has lumped together widely heterogeneous approaches to the previously described objectives of pneumostasis and pleurodesis. Great variations exist when it comes to what surgeons do inside the chest, a fact not factorised in the meta-analysis. In our opinion, it should not matter in any way or form how one enters the chest, whereas it matters what one does once inside the chest. Indeed, the Barker study showed that in studies that did the same pleurodesis through two different forms of access, the relative risk (RR) of recurrences in patients undergoing VATS compared with open surgery was similar [22].

With regard to pneumostasis, the practice varies widely between doing nothing (if a bulla is not found) and performing a variety of procedures. These include blind wedge of the lung apex (apicoectomy), ligation of bulla, tying, stitching, stapling, diathermy, applying silver nitrate and lasering among other methods [27–29]. Each of these variants might have a subgroup, for example, stapling with or without buttressing or covering the stapling line to reduce postoperative air leak. Should the treated bulla site (staple line) be covered with bioglue or a sealant agent? Which one? Does a pleural tent work? [30–32]. This choice could be an attractive option for ventilated patients in intensive care and for patients with severe secondary SP [33].

It is conceivable that some clinical importance is attached to the function of the pleura and the preservation of this function is advocated when a single apical bulla is all that explains the pneumothorax. In addition, pleurodesis is not without its complications. It can induce severe postoperative chest pain and increase the risk of bleeding and unscheduled return to theatre. In addition, it poses difficulties with subsequent thoracic surgery, e.g. if lung transplantation will be required later in life. Following this line of thinking, RCT have looked into the difference between bullectomy alone and bullectomy coupled with pleurodesis [34–36]. The general consensus, bar the Korean trial, is that pleurodesis with bullectomy reduces recurrence.

We then come to the second objective of pleurodesis. Several options exist, scratching, abrasion, partial or semitotal pleurectomy and pleural sclerosing agents [37]. Several chemical agents have been described: talc, tetracycline, minocycline, autologous blood, dextrose, etc. [38–41]. The use of chemical pleurodesis is tied to the complication of empyema, which adds insult to injury. The bottom line is that none of these techniques or agents could give a 100% guarantee of freedom from recurrence. Heterogeneity in the methodology of RCT leads to significant differences in outcomes. Nor does the meta-analysis of Barker take into account the human factor of surgical experience and learning curves. It is not useful to lump together trainees at the beginning of their VATS learning curve together with experienced surgeons in this field. Unsupervised trainees are bound to have high recurrence rates, skewing the figures. Familiarity with small details that might avert recurrence is a function of experience. Meticulous examination of the lung surfaces is vital to unveil bullae in other lobes. Seventy percent of postoperative pneumothorax recurrences probably developed because of overlooked bullae and incomplete resection of bullae in the early period of VATS experience [42]. Equally important is to scrutinise the diaphragmatic surface for fenestrations in the child-bearing age of ladies [43]. Identification of the lung margin rosary of blebs and the knowledge of how to deal with them prevent recurrence (**Figure 2**). Detailed knowledge of the stapling devices, their colour code and sizes is mandatory, as well as the realisation that the intersection point of two stapling lines is the weakest link for potential air leak. How many of us perform the bubbling test (underwater testing for air leak before and after pneumostasis)? It seems logical to make sure that there is no air leak by the end of pneumostasis, to ensure the complete expansion of the lung and guarantee pleurodesis (**Figure 3**). Many is the time we found the source of air leak hiding within an azygos lobe (**Figure 4**).

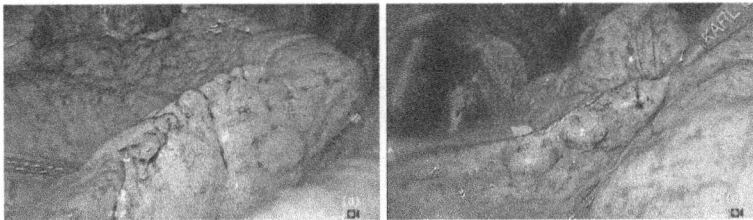

Figure 2.
(a) Rosary of marginal blebs (beads), which can lead to recurrent pneumothorax. (b) Contact diathermy obliterates them and forms a scar at the margin.

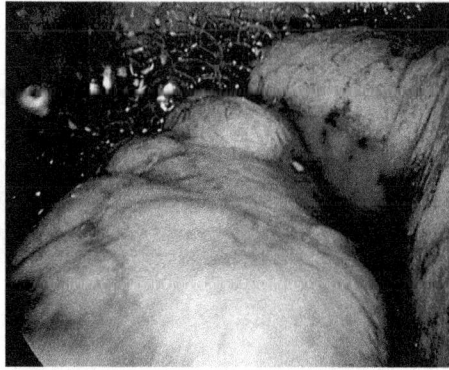

Figure 3.
Bubbling test after stapling an apical bulla. More stapling was needed until the lung was watertight.

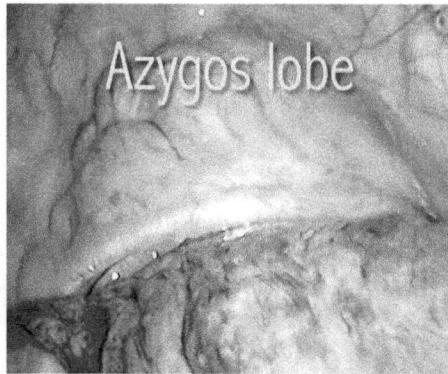

Figure 4.
Multiple apical bullae hiding within an azygos lobe.

From the above discussion, it is unreasonable to assign increased recurrence rates to the way we access the chest cavity. Access should never matter. Minimal access surgery has leapt to the forefront of access choices preferred by patients. It has proven to result in less postoperative pain, less usage of analgesics and antiemetics, early recovery, less stay in hospital and early return to work. Therefore, it is very unlikely to advocate open thoracotomy as a first-choice procedure on the basis of the previously mentioned systematic reviews alone.

5. Controversies surrounding chest drain insertion

Who should and who should not insert a chest drain? There is no consensus on this matter. However, surgical abilities even of a minor order are required to safely insert a chest drain; after all this is a surgical procedure. Therefore, proctored training is mandatory before any trainee is allowed to do it alone. Should one be certified before being allowed to perform this procedure unsupervised? This is debatable. Thoracic surgeons and their trainees are the most experienced to deal with chest drains; however, the idea that surgeons should look after all chest drains in the hospital is ludicrous and logistically unachievable.

The technique of drain insertion keeps changing. The BTS guidelines in 1993 recommend using a trocar (harpoon!); however, deaths had been reported from their use, and subsequently, the BTS changed its recommendations in an updated report in 2010 [10, 44]. Harris et al. reported on current practice and adverse incidents related to chest drains at 148 acute hospitals in the UK between 2003 and 2008 [45]. Thirty-one cases of chest drain misplacement were reported with seven deaths. Misplaced drains were inserted in the liver (10), peritoneal space (6), heart (5), spleen (5), subclavian vessels (2), colon (1), oesophagus (1) and inferior vena cava (1). One of my previous mentors at the University Hospital of Wales, the late Mr. Ian Breckenridge, has previously stated that "I regard trocar systems as potentially lethal weapons, and their misuse has been responsible for the few fatalities that I have seen, when heart, lung and liver have been lacerated" [46]. Similar serious injuries and fatalities were reported elsewhere [47–57]. Trocars are now banned from the UK. It is stating the obvious that the litigation expenses accompanying these cases are exorbitantly costly to the hospital trust and the taxpayer in the UK.

Clinicians differ about the choice of drain type and size [58]. Physicians and interventional radiologist tend to choose small calibre drains (medical drains), such as pigtails, 12F or 14F, whereas surgeons tend to put larger tubes +24F (surgical drains) [10, 59, 60]. Drain kinking, blockage and accidental dislodgment are common complications of small-bore drains (**Figure 5**). Per contra, Riber et al. in a retrospective study concluded that surgical (wide-bore) drains significantly increase the dwell time in primary SP [61]. Although they may be effective in managing pleural infection and less painful than large drains, small-bore drains may be less effective for pleurodesis [58]. The war between chest physicians and chest surgeons around the calibre of the chest drain will continue. Chest physicians have evidence that for air drainage size does not matter and a 16F drain is as good as any. Surgeons see the dysfunctional spectrum of these drains and correct the situation by inserting larger drains.

A persistent air leak with or without re-expansion of the lung is the usual reason for consideration of the use of suction, although there is no evidence for its routine use. The optimal level of suction on the drain is controversial, and so is the optimal time of its removal [62–66]. Data on the actual intrapleural pressure during the use of these systems is lacking [67]. Most of the knowledge is extrapolated from studies after lung resection, and protocols for pneumothorax drain insertion are scanty. It seems that the practice is a personal preference rather than evidence driven. We tend to believe that initial suction will guarantee the full expansion of lung and improves the chances of pleurodesis.

Recent introduction of the digital drainage systems seems to offer more physiological and dynamic mobile suction, assisting in enhanced early recovery [68, 69]. Its

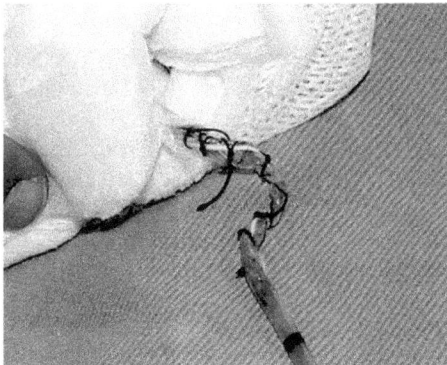

Figure 5.
Dysfunctional medical drain (14F) removed to insert a surgical drain (28F) for pneumothorax. Twisting and overtight anchorage stitch obliterated the drain lumen.

routine use has been recommended by the National Institute for Health and Clinical Excellence (NICE) after VATS pulmonary resections [70]. For how long should we leave the drain? One day, 1 week or more? Some believe (including the author) that if the drain is not serving its purpose, it should be removed. It is our practice to remove the drain the day following the surgery, provided the digital drain registers absence of air leak and the lung is fully expanded on the chest X-ray. The backdrop of such an approach is to accept reinsertion of the drain in a minority of patients when we get it wrong. The patient is allowed home after a normal chest X-ray has followed the drain removal. Others are more conservative and of the opinion that for the pleurodesis to succeed, the drain should remain in situ 3–7 days. We tend to send patients home with a Heimlich valve (flutter bag) if air leak persists more than 3 days and follow them weekly in the outpatient clinic. There are no RCTs to compare drain dwell times, and therefore general rules apply. In the absence of air leak while suction is off, and the lung is fully expanded on the chest X-ray the drain could safely be removed, otherwise; recurrence of pneumothorax is guaranteed.

There is a general consensus that drains should never be clamped [10, 71]. However, some of us do clamp drains and send patients to the radiology department for a chest X-ray, in preparation for removing the drain *despite* the air leak. It must be emphasised that this management should remain selective. This "provocative" approach in removing the drain despite air leak was described before by Kirschner et al. and Cerfolio et al. [72, 73]. If the chest X-ray shows the lung stuck to the chest wall after 2 weeks of tube time, we clamp the tube and send the patient for another X-ray. If the patient is clinically well and there is no change in lung expansion, then the drain is safely removed without bothering to close the drain site, which is usually either infected or has necrotic margins that take stitches badly. A pressure dressing is all that is needed. The stuck lung does not collapse, and the drain site closes in a week or two by secondary intention. The patient has to be reassured about the hissing sound through the drain site, which stops within a week or so.

To complicate matters further, air could entrain back into the chest at the time of drain removal. This usually leads to a small residual pneumothorax, which does not expand on subsequent radiological examination. It is important to realise the difference between erroneous drain removal and recurrence of genuine air leak. The incidence of this complication is technique-dependant and proportional to the experience of the staff member allocated for this task. Instructions given to the patient at the time of removing the drain are crucial. Again RCT about removing chest drains on full inspiration, full expiration, mid inspiration or Valsalva manoeuvre found no statistical difference, and therefore no evidence-based practice could be extrapolated [73, 74]. The rate of absorption of air in the chest is roughly 1–2% of the volume of the hemithorax every 24 hours, and complete re-expansion usually takes 2–7 weeks [75]. However, this might be too late for pleurodesis. By that time the parietal pleura (in the case of pleurectomy) would have healed, and the partially collapsed lung would not stick to the chest wall. Likewise, pleurodesing agents might be diluted or washed away by the reactive effusion, resulting in treatment failure.

From the above discussion, it is safe to conclude and agree with Lim that "No single aspect of postoperative care in general thoracic surgery is subject to more variation than the management of chest drains, … yet almost all thoracic surgeons and institutions manage chest drains differently" [76].

6. Pneumothorax and pregnancy

Spontaneous pneumothorax during pregnancy is rare but not unusual [77, 78]. Notoriously pneumothorax recurs during pregnancy and poses risks to the mother and foetus during labour. In addition, exposure to radiation of the X-rays in the first trimester is tied to foetal deformities and abnormalities. There is no unified evidence-based practice to guide management in this scenario. Historically it was managed by intercostal drainage for the rest of the pregnancy duration, thoracotomy at any stage, premature induction of labour or caesarean section. The clinician must be aware that even in the first trimester, the diaphragm moves cephalad approximately 4 cm. The classical landmarks for drain insertion do not apply.

The most contemporary recommendation of management is a conservative approach. Expectant management is recommended if the mother is not dyspnoeic and there is no foetal distress and the pneumothorax on the chest X-ray is not significant (<2 cm). Symptomatic mothers could have needle aspiration or drain insertion to resolve the pneumothorax. There is no consensus as what to do with non-resolving pneumothorax, but in our centre, we tend to assess the risk in conjunction with the obstetrician's advice and perform a VATS bullectomy and partial parietal pleurectomy. This is safe in the first trimester but should be avoided after that.

With regard to advice to the risk during labour, we adopt the one given by Lal et al. and the BTS guidelines [10, 79]. Elective-assisted delivery (forceps or ventouse extraction) at or near term is recommended, with regional (epidural) anaesthesia. Less maternal effort is required with forceps delivery, which theoretically reduces the chance of recurrence. Close cooperation between the respiratory physician, obstetrician and thoracic surgeon is essential, requiring delivery to be undertaken in a tertiary referral centre with all three specialties under one roof. If a caesarean section is unavoidable, then a spinal anaesthetic is preferable to a general anaesthetic. To avoid desaturation and tension during general anaesthesia, a prophylactic intercostal drain could be considered as a safety measure. It is advisable that the mother should undergo elective VATS procedure after convalescence due to the risk of recurrence in subsequent pregnancies.

7. Pneumothorax and air travel

Commercial air traffic is on the rise. The number of medical emergencies on-board aircraft is increasing as the age-increasing general population becomes more mobile and adventurous. Travellers with respiratory diseases are at particular risk for in-flight events. Exposure to lower atmospheric pressure in a pressurised cabin at high altitude may result in pneumothorax. Gas expansion within enclosed spaces in the human body could expand by 25–30% at the typical cruising altitude of a commercial airline flight, causing significant hypoxia. Patients at risk are those with bullae, cystic lung disease, lymphangioleiomyomatosis (LAM), pulmonary Langerhans cell histiocytosis, cystic pulmonary adenomatoid malformation (CPAM) and cystic bronchiectasis [80].

The currently available guidelines are admittedly based on sparse data and include recommendations to delay air travel for 1–3 weeks after thoracic surgery or resolution of the pneumothorax [80]. No fatalities have been reported due to pneumothorax on-board aviation generally; however, true incidence of specific illnesses associated with air travel has been difficult to assess.

The diagnosis of pneumothorax can be career limiting in the US Air Force. Once an SP has been diagnosed in an individual, he/she will be grounded from further flight duties until either 9 years have elapsed without a recurrence or there has been a bilateral parietal pleurectomy [81].

Barotrauma during or after scuba diving (also on the rise) can rarely lead to pneumothorax, especially on sudden ascent not allowing time for equilibrium. The data is sparse, and there is no solid recommendation about this sport in the literature. Snorkelling sport up to a depth of 10 m does not seem to increase the risk of pneumothorax.

8. Genetics and pneumothorax

A lot of work needs to be done in the field of spontaneous pneumothorax that runs in families. Genetic profiling in patients presenting with pneumothorax might be indicated, in the hope of finding defective genes that expose conditions such as Marfan, Ehler Danlos and Birt-Hogg-Dubé syndromes [82]. These have one thing in common, defective connective tissue. Patients may or may not have pre-existing lung cysts before their pneumothoraces, which can be bilateral and recurrent. Risk stratification of other siblings needs to be calculated and predicted [83]. The importance of this subject is realised by frequent flyers, pilots, airhostesses and scuba divers. They need to know the risk and whether prophylactic procedures would be a wise thing to go for. By the same token patients who are expected to require lung transplantation at one stage in their life, such as cystic fibrosis patients, require special consideration of treatment. Pleurodesis seems to render transplantation a difficult task, but this is not a prohibitive contraindication. It might be prudent to discuss the case with a lung transplantation centre before embarking on such treatment [84].

9. Complications of pneumothorax treatment

Getting the treatment of pneumothorax right is of paramount importance. The decision of which procedure to go for might not be crucial to fit patients but might endanger the lives of compromised patients. Patients with cardio-pulmonary compromise, severe COPD and emphysema might have very little cardiopulmonary reserve, so much so they tolerate lung collapse poorly. Air leak is known to be a killer after lung volume reduction surgery for severe COPD patients. Assessment for general anaesthesia is essential for compromised patients. Consideration of alternative local or spinal/extrapleural analgesia might be required.

Insertion of intercostal tubes under non-sterile conditions leads to infection and empyema with formation of a thick rind over the visceral pleura, trapping the lung in a collapsed position. Lung re-expansion is formidable in this scenario. Formal thoracotomy and lung decortication might be required to re-inflate the lung and prevent chronic empyema with a permanently infected cavity. We never push an intercostal drain few centimetres into the chest (as possibly suggested by the chest X-ray). Pushing a bit of the unsterile part of the tube inside the chest leads to empyema. It is, however, safe to shorten a drain by pulling it out and re-anchor it with a fresh stitch.

Severe surgical (subcutaneous) emphysema could complicate insertion of a chest drain. The clinician should be aware of the position of the last lateral holes of the tube, which should always be inside the bony chest (**Figure 6**). Until the advent of the digital systems, which tell us exactly how much air is leaking, quantifying air leak visually was a subjective bias. No leak, countable bubbles, and coalesced bubbles were the measures of air leak in the underwater seal systems. This subjective assessment leads to days of unnecessary drain dwell time. Urgency of this complication is highlighted in ventilated patients in the intensive care. Insertion of a second large intercostal drain, subcutaneous cannulae and subcutaneous small-bore drains on suction has all been tried with varying success. It should be noted that fixed wall suction in these cases might lead to tension pneumothorax and the drain must be on gravity mode without suction. Information about how to deal with surgical emphysema is very sparse, and the management of severe air leak and surgical emphysema is controversial.

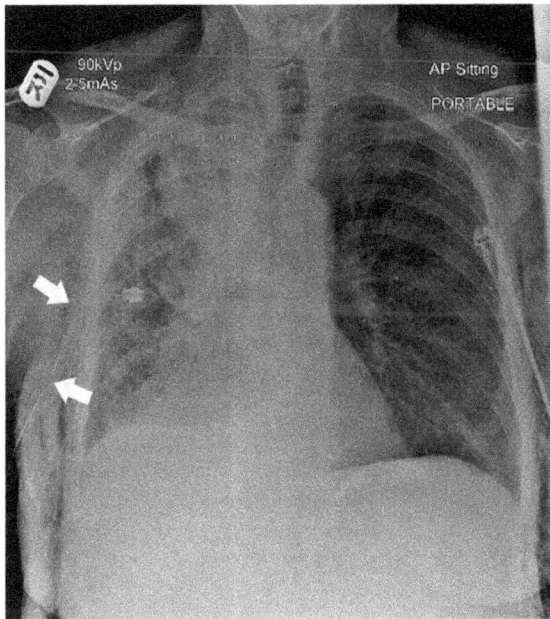

Figure 6.
Lateral holes of the intercostal drain are outside the chest, a common cause for surgical emphysema.

Should the need arise for a second drain to replace a dysfunctional one due to, e.g. blockage or kinking, the second drain should not be introduced at the site of the removed first one to reduce the risk of empyema. A fresh stab wound is better in the long run.

And last but not the least is the question of pain and analgesia which should be carefully worked out before and after surgical procedures or ward bedside pleurodesis. Talc pleurodesis is known to cause severe pain that can result in cardiac arrest, and it is, therefore, prudent to pre-empt it by administration of opioid analgesia before introducing the talcum powder or slurry [85]. The question of whether postoperative non-steroidal analgesia (NSAID) is detrimental to pleurodesis is not resolved. RCT have shown a negative predictive effect of such drugs to pleurodesis and increased incidence of recurrence. Therefore, it is best to avoid them in the immediate postoperative period [86, 87].

10. The future

There is a trend for single-port VATS procedures under sedation/epidural anaesthesia [88]. The so-called tubeless surgery has a lot to commend, avoiding the risk of general anaesthesia, early recovery and discharge from hospital. However, they have the inherent caveat of suitability for selected patients. Understanding of the technique and cooperation in case of conversion to general anaesthesia is mandatory.

Advances in diagnostic techniques have increasingly allowed the identification of lung abnormalities in patients previously labelled as having a primary spontaneous pneumothorax. This allowed different managements from that of simple pneumothorax. A good example of this is demonstrated in secondary SP. The choices for lung reduction surgery and the advent of valves have revolutionised the options for this category of severe COPD [89]. Bronchial valves have been used to treat prolonged air leak, especially in ventilated patients in the intensive care, with large air leaks and inflated lungs [90, 91]. In future we might see expansion of the use of "easily removable" and temporary bronchial valves especially in the subgroup of patients who are high risk for surgical intervention.

As the cost of VATS surgery comes down, as well as capacity increases in tertiary referral hospitals, we will see more of the operative treatment for first episode of spontaneous pneumothorax, on a semi-urgent basis (1–2 days from start of episode). Better risk stratification will identify those at high risk of recurrence and put them forward for early operation.

The economic reality of reducing cost and the technological advances might team up to drive change. It is possible to see scenarios whereby pneumothorax is treated as a day case. Patients are discharged home on the same operative day, with a chest drain in situ. They would be asked to enter the reading of air flow from the digital device daily. The information is transmitted by a social media application such as WhatsApp to the hospital which instructs the patient to call in for removal of the drain. Better still, the visiting district nurse could pay the patient a visit at home to remove the drain without the need for readmission. Fiction? Perhaps not!

Currently robotic surgery is too expensive for this type of surgery, and we have not come across any meaningful publications in this regard. However, when robotic expenses come down in due course, we might see a surge in the use of the robot.

11. Conclusion

Many controversies surround the management of pneumothorax. Surgical intervention either by VATS or open procedure leads to less incidence of recurrence. The variability in reported outcomes and the paucity of published multicentre randomised controlled trials highlight the need for further studies to investigate the best options for pneumostasis and pleurodesis.

Conflict of interest

I have previously received honoraria for providing educational material, presentations and lectures for Ethicon (Johnson & Johnson), Medtronic-Covidien and Karl Storz.

Author details

Khalid Amer
The Cardiovascular and Thoracic Centre, University Hospital Southampton NHS Foundation Trust, United Kingdom

*Address all correspondence to: khalid.amer@btinternet.com

IntechOpen

References

[1] West JB. Snorkel breathing in the elephant explains the unique anatomy of its pleura. Respiration Physiology. 2001;**126**(1):1-8

[2] Eales NB. XI—The anatomy of a Fœtal African elephant, Elephas africanus (Loxodonta africana). Part III. The contents of the thorax and abdomen, and the skeleton. Earth and Environmental Science Transactions of the Royal Society of Edinburgh. 1929;**56**(1):203-246

[3] Hartin DJ, Kendall R, Boyle AA, Atkinson PRT. Case of the month: Buffalo chest: A case of bilateral pneumothoraces due to pleuropleural communication. Emergency Medicine Journal. 2006;**23**(6):483-486

[4] Ruckley CV, McCormack RJM. The management of spontaneous pneumothorax. Thorax. 1966;**21**: 139-144

[5] Cerfolio RJ, Bryant AS. The management of chest tubes after pulmonary resection. Thoracic Surgery Clinics. 2010;**20**(3):399-405

[6] Laennec RTH. Traité du Diagnostic des Maladies des Poumons et du Coeur. Tome Second, Paris: Brosson and Chaudé; 1819. p. 4

[7] Gupta D, Hansell A, Nichols T, et al. Epidemiology of pneumothorax in England. Thorax. 2000;**55**:666-671

[8] Alifano M, Jablonski C, Kadiri H, Falcoz P, Gompel A, Camilleri-Broet S, et al. Catamenial and noncatamenial, endometriosis-related or nonendometriosis-related pneumothorax referred for surgery. American Journal of Respiratory and Critical Care Medicine. 2007;**176**:1048-1053

[9] Korom S, Canyurt H, Missbach A, et al. Catamenial pneumothorax revisited: Clinical approach and systematic review of the literature. The Journal of Thoracic and Cardiovascular Surgery. 2004;**128**:502-508

[10] MacDuff A, Arnold A, Harvey J. Management of spontaneous pneumothorax: British Thoracic Society pleural disease guideline 2010. Thorax. 2010;**65**:ii18-ii31

[11] Wilcox DT, Glick PL, Kramanoukian HL, et al. Spontaneous pneumothorax: A single institution 12-year experience in patients under 16 years of age. Journal of Pediatric Surgery. 1995;**30**:1452-1454

[12] Sadikot RT, Greene T, Meadows K, Arnold AG. Recurrence of primary spontaneous pneumothorax. Thorax. 1997;**52**(9):805-809

[13] Baumann MH, Strange C, Heffner JE, et al. AACP pneumothorax consensus group. Management of spontaneous pneumothorax: An American College of Chest Physicians Delphi consensus statement. Chest. 2001;**119**:590-602

[14] Tschopp JM, Bintcliffe O, Astoul P, Canalis E, Driesen P, Janssen J, et al. ERS task force statement: Diagnosis and treatment of primary spontaneous pneumothorax. The European Respiratory Journal. 2015;**46**(2):321-335

[15] Stradling P, Poole G. Conservative management of spontaneous pneumothorax. Thorax. 1966;**21**: 145-149

[16] Torresini G, Vaccarili M, Divisi D, Crisci R. Is video-assisted thoracic surgery justified at first spontaneous pneumothorax? European Journal of Cardio-Thoracic Surgery. 2001;**20**(1):42-45

[17] Schramel FM, Sutedja TG, Braber JC, Van Mourik JC, Postmus PE.

Cost effectiveness of video-assisted thoracoscopic surgery versus conservative treatment for first time or recurrent spontaneous pneumothorax. The European Respiratory Journal. 1996;**9**:1821-1825

[18] Al-Mourgi M, Alshehri F. Video-assisted thoracoscopic surgery for the treatment of first-time spontaneous pneumothorax versus conservative treatment. International Journal of Health Sciences. 2015;**9**(4):428-432

[19] Ooi A, Ling Z. Uniportal video assisted thoracoscopic surgery bullectomy and double pleurodesis for primary spontaneous pneumothorax. Journal of Visceral Surgery. 2016;**26**(2):17

[20] Li L, Tian H, Yue W, Li S, Gao C, Si L. Subxiphoid vs intercostal single-incision video-assisted thoracoscopic surgery for spontaneous pneumothorax: A randomised controlled trial. International Journal of Surgery. 2016;**30**:99-103

[21] Sudduth CL, Shinnick JK, Geng Z, McCracken CE, Clifton MS, Raval MV. Optimal surgical technique in spontaneous pneumothorax: A systematic review and meta-analysis. The Journal of Surgical Research. 2017;**210**:32-46

[22] Barker A, Maratos EC, Edmonds L, et al. Recurrence rates of video-assisted thoracoscopic versus open surgery in the prevention of recurrent pneumothorax: A systematic review of randomised and non-randomised trials. Lancet. 2007;**370**:329-335

[23] Sedrakyan A, van der Meulen J, Lewsey J, Treasure T. Video assisted thoracic surgery for treatment of pneumothorax and lung resections: Systematic review of randomised clinical trials. British Medical Journal. 2004;**329**(7473):1008

[24] Waller DA, Forty J, Morritt GN. Video-assisted thoracoscopic surgery versus thoracotomy for spontaneous pneumothorax. The Annals of Thoracic Surgery. 1994;**58**:372-376

[25] Ayed AK, Al-Din HJ. Video-assisted thoracoscopy versus thoracotomy for primary spontaneous pneumothorax: A randomized controlled trial. Medical Principles and Practice. 2000;**9**:113-118

[26] Vohra HA, Adamson L, Weeden DF. Does video-assisted thoracoscopic pleurectomy result in better outcomes than open pleurectomy for primary spontaneous pneumothorax? Interactive Cardiovascular and Thoracic Surgery. 2008;**7**:673-677

[27] LoCicero J, Hartz RS, Frederikson JW, et al. New applications of laser in pulmonary surgery (hemostasis and sealing of air leaks). The Annals of Thoracic Surgery. 1985;**40**:546-550

[28] Marcheix B, Brouchet L, Renaud C, et al. Videothoracoscopic silver nitrate pleurodesis for primary spontaneous pneumothorax: An alternative to pleurectomy and pleural abrasion? European Journal of Cardio-Thoracic Surgery. 2007;**31**(6):1106-1109. DOI: 10.1016/j.ejcts.2007.03.017

[29] Potaris K, Mihos P, Gakidis I. Experience with an albumin-glutaraldehyde tissue adhesive in sealing air leaks after bullectomy. The Heart Surgery Forum. 2003;**6**(5):429-433

[30] Matar AF, Hill JG, Duncan W, et al. Use of biological glue to control pulmonary air leaks. Thorax. 1990;**45**:670-674

[31] Hong KP, Kim DK, Kang KH. Staple line coverage with a polyglycolic acid patch and fibrin glue without pleural abrasion after thoracoscopic bullectomy for primary spontaneous pneumothorax. Korean Journal of

Thoracic and Cardiovascular Surgery. 2016;**49**(2):85-91

[32] Lee S, Kim HR, Cho S, Huh DM, Lee EB, Ryu KM, et al. Korean pneumothorax study group. Staple line coverage after bullectomy for primary spontaneous pneumothorax: A randomized trial. The Annals of Thoracic Surgery. 2014;**98**(6):2005-2011

[33] Nicotera SP, Decamp MM. Special situations: Air leak after lung volume reduction surgery and in ventilated patients. Thoracic Surgery Clinics. 2010;**20**(3):427-434

[34] Ferguson LJ, Imrie CW, Hutchison J. Excision of bullae without pleurectomy in patients with spontaneous pneumothorax. The British Journal of Surgery. 1981;**68**:214-216

[35] Horio H, Nomori H, Kobayashi R, Naruke T, Suemasu K. Impact of additional pleurodesis in video-assisted thoracoscopic bullectomy for primary spontaneous pneumothorax. Surgical Endoscopy. 2002;**16**(4):630-634

[36] Nakanishi K. Long-term effect of a thoracoscopic stapled bullectomy alone for preventing the recurrence of primary spontaneous pneumothorax. Surgery Today. 2009;**39**(7):553-557

[37] Min X, Huang Y, Yang Y, Chen Y, Cui J, Wang C, et al. Mechanical pleurodesis does not reduce recurrence of spontaneous pneumothorax: A randomized trial. The Annals of Thoracic Surgery. 2014;**98**(5):1790-1796

[38] Chung WJ, Jo W, Lee SH, Son HS, Kim KT. Effects of additional pleurodesis with dextrose and talc-dextrose solution after video assisted thoracoscopic procedures for primary spontaneous pneumothorax. Journal of Korean Medical Science. 2008;**23**(2):284-287

[39] Hallifax RJ, Yousuf A, Jones HE, et al. Effectiveness of chemical pleurodesis in spontaneous pneumothorax recurrence prevention: A systematic review. Thorax. 2017;**72**:1121-1131

[40] Shackcloth MJ, Poullis M, Jackson M, Soorae A, Page RD. Intrapleural instillation of autologous blood in the treatment of prolonged air leak after lobectomy: A prospective randomized controlled trial. The Annals of Thoracic Surgery. 2006;**82**(3):1052-1056

[41] Milanez JR, Vargas FS, Filomeno LT, et al. Intrapleural talc for prevention of recurrent pneumothorax. Chest. 1994;**106**:1162-1165

[42] Haraguchi S, Koizumi K, Hioki M, Orii K, Kinoshita H, Endo N, et al. Postoperative recurrences of pneumothorax in video-assisted thoracoscopic surgery for primary spontaneous pneumothorax in young patients. Journal of Nippon Medical School. 2008;**75**(2):91-95

[43] Cowl CT, Dunn WF, Deschamps C. Visualisations of diaphragmatic fenestration associated with catamenial pneumothorax. The Annals of Thoracic Surgery. 1999;**68**:1413-1414

[44] Miller AC, Harvey JE. Guidelines for management of spontaneous pneumothorax. Standards of care committee, British Thoracic Society. British Medical Journal. 1993;**307**:114-116

[45] Harris A, O'Driscoll BR, Turkington PM. Survey of major complications of intercostal chest drain insertion in the UK. Postgraduate Medical Journal. 2010;**86**:68-72

[46] Breckenridge IM. Risk management of chest drains. Clinical Risk. 2001;**7**:91-93

[47] Haggie JA. Management of pneumothorax. Chest drain trocar unsafe and unnecessary. British Medical

Journal. 1993;**307**:443. DOI: 10.1136/bmj.307.6901.443

[48] Kwiatt M, Tarbox A, Seamon MJ, et al. Thoracostomy tubes: A comprehensive review of complications and related topics. International Journal of Critical Illness and Injury Science. 2014;**4**(2):143-155

[49] Tait P, Waheed U, Bell S. Successful removal of malpositioned chest drain within the liver by embolization of the transhepatic track. Cardiovascular and Interventional Radiology. 2009;**32**:825-827

[50] Osinowo O, Softah AL, Eid Zahrani M. Ectopic chest tube insertions: Diagnosis and strategies for prevention. The African Journal of Medical Sciences. 2002;**31**:67-70

[51] Nahum E, Ben-Ari J, Schonfeld T, Horev G. Acute diaphragmatic paralysis caused by chest-tube trauma to phrenic nerve. Pediatric Radiology. 2001;**31**:444-446

[52] Taub PJ, Lajam F, Kim U. Erosion into the subclavian artery by a chest tube. The Journal of Trauma. 1999;**47**:972-974

[53] Knyazer B et al. Horner's syndrome secondary to chest tube insertion for pneumothorax. Asian Journal of Ophthalmology. 2008;**10**:27-29

[54] Etoch SW, Bar-Natan MF, Miller FB, Richardson JD. Tube thoracostomy. Factors related to complications. Archives of Surgery. 1995;**130**:521-525. Discussion 525-6

[55] Banagale RC, Outerbridge EW, Aranda JV. Lung perforation: A complication of chest tube insertion in neonatal pneumothorax. The Journal of Pediatrics. 1979;**94**:973-975

[56] Icoz G, Kara E, Ilkgül O, Yetgin S, Tunçyürek P, Korkut MA. Perforation of the stomach due to chest tube complication in a patient with iatrogenic diaphragmatic rupture. Acta Chirurgica Belgica. 2003;**103**:423-424

[57] Johnson JF, Wright DR. Chest tube perforation of esophagus following repair of esophageal atresia. Journal of Pediatric Surgery. 1990;**25**:1227-1230

[58] Hallifax RJ, Psallidas I, Rahman NM. Chest drain size: The debate continues. Current Pulmonology Reports. 2017;**6**(1):26-29

[59] Fang M, Liu G, Luo G, Wu T. Does pigtail catheters relieve pneumothorax? A PRISMA-compliant systematic review and meta-analysis. Medicine. 2018;**97**(47):89

[60] Filosso PL, Sandri A, Guerrera F, Ferraris A, Marchisio F, Bora G, et al. When size matters: Changing opinion in the management of pleural space-the rise of small-bore pleural catheters. Journal of Thoracic Disease. 2016;**8**(7):E503-E510

[61] Riber SS, Riber LP, Olesen WH, Licht PB. The influence of chest tube size and position in primary spontaneous pneumothorax. Journal of Thoracic Disease. 2017;**9**(2):327-332

[62] Sharma TN, Agrihotri SP, Jain NK, et al. Intercostal tube thoracostomy in pneumothorax: Factors influencing re-expansion of lung. The Indian Journal of Chest Diseases & Allied Sciences. 1988;**30**:32-35

[63] Reed MF, Lyons JM, Luchette FA, et al. Preliminary report of a prospective, randomized trial of underwater seal for spontaneous and iatrogenic pneumothorax. Journal of the American College of Surgeons. 2007;**204**:84-90

[64] Blair Marshall M, Deeb ME, Bleier J, Kucharczuk JC, Friedberg JS, Kaiser LR, et al. Suction vs water

seal after pulmonary resection. Chest. 2002;**121**(3):831-835

[65] Cerfolio RJ, Bass C, Katholi CR. Prospective randomized trial compares suction versus water seal for air leaks. The Annals of Thoracic Surgery. 2001;**71**(5):1613-1617

[66] SY S, DY Y. Catheter drainage of spontaneous pneumothorax: Suction or no suction, early or late removal? Thorax. 1982;**37**:46-48

[67] Aguayo E, Cameron R, Dobaria V, Ou R, Iyengar A, Sanaiha Y, et al. Assessment of differential pressures in chest drainage systems: Is what you see what you get? The Journal of Surgical Research. 2018;**232**:464-469

[68] Pompili C, Detterbeck F, Papagiannopoulos K, Sihoe A, Vachlas K, Maxfield MW, et al. Multicenter international randomized comparison of objective and subjective outcomes between electronic and traditional chest drainage systems. The Annals of Thoracic Surgery. 2014;**98**(2):490-496

[69] Gilbert S, McGuire AL, Maghera S, Sundaresan SR, Seely AJ, Maziak DE, et al. Randomized trial of digital versus analog pleural drainage in patients with or without a pulmonary air leak after lung resection. The Journal of Thoracic and Cardiovascular Surgery. 2015;**150**:1243-1249

[70] Thopaz+ Portable Digital System for Managing Chest Drains. NICE. 2018. Available from: https://www.nice.org.uk/guidance/MTG37/chapter/1-Recommendations [Accessed: November 11, 2018]

[71] Wong PS. Management of pneumothorax. Never clamp a chest drain. British Medical Journal. 1993;**307**:443

[72] Kirschner PA. "Provocative clamping" and removal of chest tubes despite persistent air leak. The Annals of Thoracic Surgery. 1992;**53**:740-741

[73] Cerfolio RJ, Minnich DJ, Bryant AS. The removal of chest tubes despite an air leak or a pneumothorax. The Annals of Thoracic Surgery. 2009;**87**:1690-1694

[74] Bell RL, Ovadia P, Abdullah F, Spector S, Rabinovici R. Chest tube removal: End-inspiration or end-expiration? The Journal of Trauma. 2001;**50**(4):674-677

[75] Novoa NM, Jiménez MF, Varela G. When to remove a chest tube. Thoracic Surgery Clinics. 2017;**27**(1):41-46

[76] Lim E. The devil is in the details: Managing chest drains and interpreting negative randomized trial data. The Journal of Thoracic and Cardiovascular Surgery. 2015;**150**:1252-1253

[77] Traoré A, Doumiri M, Bensghir M, Haimeur C, Tazi AS. Management of spontaneous pneumothorax during pregnancy: A case report and review of literature. Revue de Pneumologie Clinique. 2015;**71**(5):306-308

[78] Terndrup TE, Bosco SF, McLean ER. Spontaneous pneumothorax complicating pregnancy: Case report and review of the literature. The Journal of Emergency Medicine. 1989;**7**:245-248

[79] Lal A, Anderson G, Cowen M, et al. Pneumothorax and pregnancy. Chest. 2007;**132**:1044-1048

[80] Hu X, Cowl CT, Baqir M, Ryu MJ. Air travel and pneumothorax. Chest. 2014;**145**(4):688-694

[81] Voge VM, Anthracite R. Spontaneous pneumothorax in the USAF aircrew population: A retrospective study. Aviation, Space, and Environmental Medicine. 1986;**57**:939-949

[82] Gupta N, Sunwoo BY, Kotloff RM. Birt-Hogg-Dubé syndrome. Clinics in Chest Medicine. 2016;**37**(3):475-486

[83] Viveiro C, Rocha P, Carvalho C, et al. Spontaneous pneumothorax as manifestation of Marfan syndrome. BMJ Case Reports. 2013;**2013**:pii: bcr2013201697

[84] Weill D. Lung transplantation: Indications and contraindications. Journal of Thoracic Disease. 2018;**10**(7):4574-4587

[85] Tschopp JM, Boutin C, Astoul P, Janssen JP, Grandin S, Bolliger CT, et al. Talcage by medical thoracoscopy for primary spontaneous pneumo-thorax is more cost-effective than drainage: A randomised study. The European Respiratory Journal. 2002;**20**:1003-1009

[86] Ben-Nun A, Golan N, Faibishenko I, Simansky D, Soudack M. Nonsteroidal anti-inflammatory medications: Efficient and safe treatment following video-assisted pleurodesis for spontaneous pneumothorax. World Journal of Surgery. 2011;**35**(11):2563-2567

[87] Lardinois D, Vogt P, Yang L, Hegyi I, Baslam M, Weder W. Non-steroidal anti-inflammatory drugs decrease the quality of pleurodesis after mechanical pleural abrasion. European Journal of Cardio-Thoracic Surgery. 2004;**25**(5):865-871

[88] Pompeo E, Tacconi F, Mineo D, Mineo TC. The role of awake video-assisted thoracoscopic surgery in spontaneous pneumothorax. The Journal of Thoracic and Cardiovascular Surgery. 2007;**133**(3):786-790

[89] Kemp SV, Herth FJF, Shah PL. Bullectomy: A waste of space or room for improvement? Respiration. 2016;**92**:218-219

[90] Keshishyan S, Revelo AE, Epelbaum O. Bronchoscopic management of prolonged air leak. Journal of Thoracic Disease. 2017;**9**(Suppl 10):S1034-S1046

[91] Wood DE, Cerfolio RJ, Gonzalez X, Springmeyer SC. Bronchoscopic management of prolonged air leak. Clinics in Chest Medicine. 2010;**31**(1):127-133